Facing Up To It
a triumphant memoir

Dawn Shaw

Published by Facing Up to It

Copyright 2012 Dawn Shaw
A Facing Up to It Publication

First Published by Journey Grrrl Publishing, 2012
Washington, DC

Second Edition: Published by Facing Up to It, 2017
Grapeview, WA

All rights reserved.

ISBN: 978-0-692-83386-5

DISCLAIMER

No part of this publication may be reproduced or transmitted in any form or by any means, mechanical or electronic, including photocopying or recording, or by any information storage and retrieval system, or transmitted by email without permission in writing from the author. Reviewers may quote brief passages in reviews.

Neither the author nor the publisher assumes any responsibility for errors, omissions, or contrary interpretations of the subject matter herein. Any perceived slight of any individual or organization is purely unintentional.

Cover Design: Carolyn Sheltraw
Original cover concept by Drai Bearwomyn
Cover Photos by Dawn Shaw and AJC Photography
Back Cover Photo by Barry Gregg
Internal Design: Carolyn Sheltraw
Editor: Debra Ginsberg
Author's photo courtesy of the author, taken by AJC Photography.

Mother and Father

It couldn't have been easy raising

a child with a facial difference,

but there are far more challenging scenarios.

I Love You

My mother passed away one month

after initial publication.

I miss her every day.

"Scene after scene passes by my life.

The window's a wound,

The road is a knife.

The irony, ask me

"Where have you been?"

I don't know

I don't know

Because I don't know where to begin."

from *One Prairie Outpost*
Courtesy of Carbon Leaf
Lyrics by Barry Privett
www.carbonleaf.com

Table of Contents

Prologue – p. ix
1. Two Brains?
2. The Reshaping of Me
3. Protected
4. Third of Three
5. My Place in the Herd
6. Reconstruction
7. Aftermath
8. Wired
9. When Wishes Are Horses
10. Setbacks
11. Here There Be Dragons
12. The Bitter Suffering of Success
13. Distractions and Motivations
14. My Choice to Make
15. Dancing 'Round the Fire
16. Rough-Shod
17. With Great Resolution
18. The Long Haul
19. Activity as Tolerated
20. Alone in a Crowded Room
21. Academic Pursuits
22. Backstage in Black
23. Restoration
24. Images
25. Depictions
26. Empathy
27. Solitude
28. Epic Fail
29. With Great Resolve
30. Expressions
31. The Kindness of Strangers
32. Presentation
33. Burning Candles and Getting Burned
34. But I'm Not…
35. Taking Flight
36. Continuing Education
37. Emotional Spin-Dry
38. Another Woman's Man
39. Jigger
40. Walking Through a Storm
41. Wake Up Call
42. A Man of My Own
43. Electric Circus
44. Lighting Up the Stage
45. Down Under
46. Learning Curves
47. Career Moves
48. The Source
49. Silver Linings
50. A Part of Something
51. The Cuckoo's Mire
52. An Education
53. An American in Iceland
54. Humble Pie
55. Moments of Truth
56. Being Unforgettable
57. With the Band
58. Out of Sight, Out of Mind

Resources – p. 340
Acknowledgements – p. 342
About the Author – p. 343
Thank You Offer – p. 344

Prologue
My Reflection

The air is heavy and cold on a winter's day as I return home from a ride on one of the many Icelandic horses I keep on my small farm. His shoes clink against gravel, displacing small rocks with each stride. My legs are warm against the saddle, gloved hands grip the reins, and my riding helmet crowns me snuggly, shielding my head from the chill. I am relieved that the rain has held off. As we near my driveway, I hear the distinctive putter of a diesel engine approaching. It's the same boxy white truck which had passed us previously, and now it's on its way out.

I rein the wooly beast into my driveway and we face the truck, waiting for it to pass. It is a rule of mine on rides that I always pass the driveway coming home so the horse doesn't get too excited about bee-lining to the barn, so after the behemoth rumbles past, we follow in its odorous wake.

Just ahead of us, the truck pulls off the road, parking in a turn-around intended for county maintenance vehicles. I watch curiously, halting the horse, wondering what the driver is up to. He climbs out of the cab and approaches me.

"Can I ask you a stupid question?" he asks.

My first thought is that he's going to ask for directions, though I'm not sure how that qualifies as stupid.

"Sure, you can ask but I'm not sure I'll have an answer," I reply.

"Is your name Dawn?" he queries.

I draw in my breath. Certainly not the question I expected. *Of course I know the answer to that question. Where does he know me from?*

"Yeah, it is," I say cautiously. I search his features, struggling for any sign of recognition, but he is not at all familiar to me.

"I think I knew you in elementary school. In Poulsbo?" He offers his name. No bells ring.

I sigh. Apprehension and the feeling I should know this guy are replaced by dry amusement. *Here we go again.*

"Um, yeah, could be. I did go there." I feign bewilderment, but I am certain his recognition is accurate. And the reason gushes into my consciousness like a flash flood.

After all this time and all I've been through, has my face really not changed that much?

Further conversation reveals that he knew me in possibly the 3rd grade and he remembers accurately that I had a lot of braces on my teeth. His name is not familiar to me at all. He didn't know me very long because his parents divorced and he moved and changed schools. Despite our brief co-existence, not only does he remember my face but my name as well. He insists that he has a good memory for faces, but I can tell he's trying to be polite. We were eight years old and weren't even in the same class, and it's been a long time. I consider myself securely off the hook for not remembering him.

This meeting is not an isolated incident. Periodically, people start conversations with me, fully expecting me to know who they are because they remember the details of our acquaintance quite clearly. Meanwhile, I am wracking my brains in frustration, trying to place them and feeling guilty for not remembering who they are. All the while I'm trying to hold a polite conversation until they either catch on that I have no clue and volunteer the information; I blunder through the conversation and we both move on; or I awkwardly come out and ask them how they know me.

These encounters offer acute reminders that I have a face others tend not to forget.

Mirror, Mirror, on the wall. Who's the fairest of them all?
I am not characterized by an attractive face.

"Beauty is only skin deep." "It's what's inside that counts." All my life, cliché after cliché ricocheted around my brain. Maybe I even believed some of them. But what's inside is flesh, blood and bone, like everyone else. OK, not quite like everyone else. Some of it has been removed or rearranged.

And I have character flaws. Like everyone else.

My reflection is broken, as in a mirror cracked. It is distorted, as in a carnival fun house. But it is not horrifying, nor would I consider it ugly. What it lacks in symmetry it makes up for in expression. It is unique, and it has shaped my life in ways I have only begun to understand.

The reflection is me.

Chapter One
Two Brains?

"What is it? What's wrong?" my mother demands, her exhaustion from birthing her third child forgotten as the staff mobilizes hurriedly from routine delivery to medical emergency. There's hardly even a chance to utter "it's a girl!"

It is August 23, 1966 in a Seattle, Washington hospital. My frantic mother is Adrienne Daugherty, originally from New York and currently a homemaker. My father, Richard Daugherty, rushes to her side as the miracle of birth quickly becomes a nightmare, his face betraying concern akin to fear. He is an electrical engineer and civil servant working for the Alaska Communications System, but a native Washingtonian.

What has become immediately apparent to those on the receiving end as I emerge is that I seem to have two heads. No, not two heads, but rather a significant fleshy lump protruding from the left side of my face. It stretches my brand new skin to unimaginable limits and I am struggling to breathe.

I am whisked away so that an immediate tracheostomy can be performed, out of sight of my confused and anxious parents. Knowing only that I have a breathing obstruction, they have granted permission for a tube to be inserted into my windpipe at the base of my throat, thus bypassing the obstruction and facilitating my breathing. But they don't understand what is actually wrong. No one does. Only after this life-saving procedure do my parents get a good look at me.

My father describes the potentially lethal lump as being as large as his fist. Since my father is approximately 6'4" tall and of a strong and sturdy build with hands to match, it is not unreasonable to assume that this protrusion is probably close to the same size as my entire, and assuredly singular, head.

I am transferred within hours to a children's hospital, where I spend the majority of the first five months of my life, and where my worried mother, once recovered from the otherwise uncomplicated delivery, spends much of the next five months of hers.

Somewhere among the waiting and the chaos, the name Dawn Carol Daugherty is scribed onto my birth certificate.

The day following my delivery, my condition has stabilized, so the doctors embark on a quest to determine just what this protrusion is made of. It is primarily on the left side of my neck, extending forward from the bone just behind my ear, protruding above and below the lower jaw and pushing my ear upward. My windpipe and voice box have also been shoved to one side. It seems by all appearances to be a large cyst with a very thick wall. The material contained therein, however, is not cystic fluid. Another large, firm mass extends beneath my tongue, behind my voice box, and all the way across the floor of my mouth toward my right jaw. Blood vessels are stretched out over the top of it, and my facial nerve is above it and not involved. My left carotid artery, which supplies oxygen to the brain, and my jugular are displaced and very thinned out. Given the threat to my brain's blood and oxygen supply, I consider myself lucky I don't have brain damage.

The surgical team does its best to thoroughly shell out the mysterious contents, not unlike a child using a large metal spoon to extract the seeds and pulp from a Halloween pumpkin. However, since the left side of my neck and face is essentially being held up by this intrusion, they leave some of the inner lining to aid in continued support of my neck. My skin, stretched considerably by the bulging mass, falls slack into a large fold. Natural growth will eventually fill this in.

After careful study of samples of the tissue removed from the site, the pathology report identifies the mass as *Benign Cervical Teratoma*.

A teratoma is a rapidly growing variety of tumor, generally composed of tissue from varying parts of the body, such as the brain, bone, cartilage, skin, lung and gastrointestinal tract that have somehow collected in a unified but unorganized mass.

The primary content of mine is brain tissue. So instead of two heads, I seem to have two brains. Or at least a bunch of extra brain tissue. *Does this make me smarter?*

My parents recall being told there are only 39 known cases in medical history. I must be quite the spectacle.

Personal research indicates that there are now over 150 known cases of congenital cervical teratoma, which make up less than 0.1% of all tumors observed in children. While such tumors are characteristically benign, mortality results from obstructed airways, causing breathing and respiratory distress. In my case, while impaired, my breathing had been sufficient to keep me alive until the tracheostomy could be performed.

My mother comes regularly to visit me, donning the white gown necessary for visits to the intensive care unit where I am under constant observation. She carries me around tenderly, lovingly nurturing the mother-child bond, torn by all-too-frequent separation. When she is not there, I am often held by the nurses. I am by no means ignored, neglected or starved for touch and attention.

On November 8, 1966, now armed with the knowledge of what they are dealing with, the doctors operate to excise the tumor. Considering my age and size, this is a delicate procedure. They remove it by dissection, carefully working around bone structure, nerves, veins, arteries and blood vessels. Microscopic examination of removed tissue reveals no malignancy present.

I am discharged from the hospital on November 21st. At nearly 3 months of age, I am transported home for the first time to meet my two older siblings.

The oldest is my brother Brian, who has recently turned four and is starting preschool. The middle child is my sister Lynne, whose earliest memory is of being dropped suddenly at the home of a family friend while my parents rush to the hospital to attend to some medical emergency I am experiencing. She is two and wonders why she hasn't met me yet. Despite the emotional drain of having me in the hospital, my mother devotes equal time to them. They are neither forgotten nor neglected, though I imagine at times they feel that way.

My parents are fortunate to have a great support system. My paternal grandmother lives reasonably close so Brian and Lynne often stay with her while my mother is spending time with me or subsequently taking me to endless doctor appointments. Family friends and women from my mother's church fill in when necessary. My father works, earning the money to support the family. The insurance benefits through his government job absorb the majority of what must be extraordinary medical bills, allowing the family to maintain the comforts of a middle class lifestyle, as I am indeed an expensive child.

But being the breadwinner has its downside. He is not as present in my life as my mother is. The doctors barely know him, yet my mother is met consistently with warm recognition. It is not because he doesn't care. His role is different, and he is there when he needs to be, as my parents' long standing marriage will testify.

Chapter Two
The Reshaping of Me

Apparently this tumor is tenacious and is not going to give in without a fight. Just over a month later and two short days after Christmas, I am readmitted to the children's hospital where the doctors discover that the tumor has defiantly grown back.

On January 3, 1967 the surgeons attack again in a two-part assault to rid me of the foe once and for all. My parents sit fretfully, awaiting news, distracted from their concern only by my bored, uncomprehending siblings trying in vain to amuse themselves in the hospital waiting room.

When the surgeons open the old incision, cutting parallel to my jaw line, they find a gleaming white mass just like its predecessor. While smaller than before, it is still of significant size.

During part one of this procedure, the surgeons are more precise, confining their incisions carefully below my facial nerve. They remove most of the newly grown tumor, leaving only a small portion at the base of the tongue.

Each step of the way, my parents are involved in the decision-making process. Not that there are many options presented, but for what they are about to do, the medical staff needs the consent forms signed.

The next procedure will reshape my face and profoundly affect the rest of my life. Whether my parents understand this fully at the time hardly matters. They agree to what is necessary to save my life.

When the surgical team goes back in for the rest of the tumor just over two weeks later for part two, they are not able to be so careful and delicate. Their effort begins with a new incision which splits my lip and runs down the left side of my chin, adding another permanent scar to my increasing collection.

In order to excise the tumor once and for all, the surgeons are forced to remove parts of my jawbone, muscle and facial nerve. These are fundamental parts of my facial structure which I will come to miss greatly later on. The front of my jaw where the teeth grow remains, but now it is anchored only by the jaw structure on the right side. The left side becomes free-floating.

A pathologist present at the surgery examines each piece that is removed to be sure there is no residual tumor. All test negative, or tumor-free, except for one tiny 6 mm area near the base of my skull. However, the surgeons are unable to do anything more at that particular site given its delicate location, so they close up and hope for the best.

The pathologist's report indicates for the first time that the tumor is potentially malignant. Cancer. They cannot be certain they have removed it all, or how it might manifest in the future.

So for this tiny child, now permanently misshapen, the future is still uncertain. I am barely visible amongst the tubes and monitoring wires, steadfastly clinging to life as I have from the beginning. Only the stubborn survive these repeated assaults. All reports indicate that I tolerate the procedures well, often awake before leaving the operating table. I am a quiet baby. I don't think it's possible to cry through a tracheostomy tube, though I'm sure I tried.

I am discharged on February 4th, 1967, not even five months old.

This time the surgeons have won; the enemy vanquished. No cancer treatments are necessary, and no cancer returns. But now pieces are missing. On an infant, such pieces are small, but as what remains grows along with the living being, the gaps grow as well. The left side of my face is mostly paralyzed and permanently numb from severed nerves. I suffer considerable hearing loss in my left ear. I never experience my mother's breast or even the rubber nipple of a baby bottle. I am no longer able to control the muscles that allow me to seal my mouth around such an object and suckle. When I am no longer fed with a tube, I drink from a cup. Even that is a challenge.

As my survival seems more assured and the tumor's demise more certain, the arduous task of trying to rebuild begins.

In November of that same year, my doctor grafts new bone onto my left jaw to partially replace what was removed. The pathology report indicates that there is no evidence of teratoma at this time. In fact, there is no evidence of foreign matter at all, and areas of missing bone have been replaced by soft tissue.

The bone graft is inserted through the existing scar site along the jaw line. It is locked into place with wire sutures. I still require a tracheostomy to facilitate breathing during surgery, but it is able to be removed immediately after the procedure. The tracheostomy scar takes the form of an indentation at the base of my throat, and remains as a lifelong reminder.

Aside from frequent check-ups and x-rays, I am left in the sole care of my family for over a year. In December of 1968 at the age of two, I am admitted to the hospital for the fourth time, this time to insert a *Silastic*, or medical grade plastic implant, in an attempt to restore the contours of the left side of my face.

The implant is wired into place without difficulty and I am sent home two days after surgery, thus setting a new record for my shortest hospital stay ever. However, the implant proves unsuccessful and is removed by the time I turn four.

Before I come to realize that I entered the world with the tumor already protruding from my cheek and neck, I'd hoped there might exist a photograph of me taken shortly after birth which would show a normal, healthy baby. That perhaps I'd had a fleeting moment of normalcy before the rapidly growing tumor and subsequent removal ravaged my features forever. I am disappointed to learn that no such photo exists, because the opportunity was never there for one to be taken.

Chapter Three
Protected

Perhaps I am drawn to animals as a toddler because my appearance doesn't matter to them. Animals are honest. The contented purr of a cat, the enthusiastic wag of a dog's tail, and the welcoming nicker of a horse are obvious signs that they are happy to interact with me. There is no hidden agenda. When an animal looks at me, it assesses my relative position, the speed of my movements, and my body language. It doesn't regard me any differently from any other human.

When a person looks at me, the first thing he or she notices is that my face doesn't line up quite right. Because people are drawn by things in our environment that stand out as unusual, my face attracts unwanted attention.

While most adults try to be discreet, children will often rivet their gazes on me in fascination. I don't remember much from my early childhood, but I do remember encounters with curious children, and my father's reaction.

We are on the ferry to Seattle. I am maybe 9 at the time, and my whole family is in one of the booths in the central section that has a table. The boat is moving, gliding across Puget Sound with a low rumble, sometimes vibrating the table so it hums. I'm sitting on the outside edge of the padded bench, looking at a picture book. My sister Lynne is playing solitaire. My mother, who is sitting next to me, and Brian are both reading. My dad is sitting across from me, and I see him bristle and his face becomes hard. He is glaring and I follow his gaze to a little girl whom he has caught staring at me. I feel the familiar sting of this hurtful reminder.

"It's not polite to stare," he growls at the child, causing her to look away and scramble behind an adult seated nearby, probably her mother. The mother looks at her daughter, who points at us wordlessly. The mom quickly assesses the situation, glancing from my face to my dad's. My father is an intimidating man when he wants to be, and his protectiveness of me has a fierce edge to it, but he looks away rather than confront her. Like most parents in similar situations, she does not challenge him. Perhaps she pities him for having to raise such a child.

Her curiosity unquenched, the child peeks around from behind her parent, stealing glances at me. No one else seems to notice this except me, so I turn away, ashamed, hoping that if my face is hidden the girl will have nothing to stare at.

In the corner of my vision, the girl appears again. She has moved around the table to get a better view of me. I turn once again, frustrated, this time facing my father.

"She's still staring at me," I complain.

He stands up threateningly, but doesn't change position. My whole family is watching now.

"Richard…" my mom starts, as if concerned he might actually do something.

Meanwhile, the girl's mother grabs her hand and leads her back to their seat, speaking quietly to her daughter and sending an apologetic look toward my parents.

My family resumes normal activity, but it takes awhile for the consuming hurt I'm feeling to dissipate.

My father's protective responses make me feel loved. Even if the cause of the attention is negative, it is attention and sometimes I instigate his support by helping him to notice offenders. But ultimately his reactions serve to make me more defensive, and in time I start offering sharp, angry responses of my own.

My parents' protectiveness extends to making sure that my jaw, which is fragile due to not being securely anchored to my skull, isn't damaged further. Not far from our house in Edmonds, a boy my age lives with his grandparents. For a short while, he and I are playmates. I am not much into "girly" stuff like dolls anyway, so I am happy to play with toy cars. However, the boy proves to be a rough companion. One day, for no apparent reason, he slams a door in my face as I am coming up the stairs behind him. No worse damage is done other than knocking out a baby tooth, but the surprise and pain starts me crying. His grandparents call my parents, who come collect their wailing child. Once recovered from this incident, I don't understand why they won't let me play with him anymore. When they tell me it's because they're afraid he might hurt me, I don't understand their concern.

I don't have many friends, especially ones so close and convenient. I miss the interaction, and I miss the toys we played with. I am hungry for acceptance by children my own age. He accepted me and I don't remember him making an issue of my appearance. I certainly didn't notice if he was troubled in other ways. My parents pull me out of what they consider a potentially dangerous situation. I am too young to recognize that acceptance at any cost is what sucks needy people into harmful relationships.

In the summer of 1972, my dad's job takes us all to Titusville, Florida. He is employed at the time by the Naval Torpedo Station in Keyport, Washington, but Titusville is the home of a major portion of the space program and one of the launch facilities in this region of Florida has been converted over to fleet support for torpedo testing.

I don't have much opinion about the move since I am only just turning six and really don't understand what all this relocation stuff means. I am sad to leave what friends I have behind and apprehensive about starting a new school where I don't know anyone.

"You'll make new friends," I am told.

I begin the first grade there at age six, but much of the material being taught to my class is already familiar.

We sit in the reading circle, our *Dick and Jane* texts open on our laps. The large double-spaced type stares up at me as I wait impatiently for my turn to read.

"Dick — and — Spot — wa—lk to. the. park…"

The kid next to me is reading so haltingly I have to resist the urge to jump in and read it for him. This would get me in trouble with the teacher and I don't want that. He struggles through another couple of sentences.

"That's very good," praises the teacher. *No it's not, thinks I.* "Now Dawn, read the next paragraph."

I breeze through the next four sentences with hardly a hesitation, eagerly showing off my superior skills. *This is how it's done,* I think with smug satisfaction. I look up at the teacher, my eyes pleading her to allow me to continue. But she calls on the next child to take her turn.

My mom tells me that the difference is in the school system. What I learned in pre-school back in Washington is what is taught in the first grade here. It also helps that my mother reads to me almost every night, enhancing my reading and listening skills.

My teacher gives me extra assignments in an effort to challenge me. I am given maps to read but I don't find them to be much of a challenge at all. This makes me feel superior and smart. If I am treated differently by the other kids I've long since repressed those memories. Nor do I remember having many school friends either.

Outside of school, however, I have friends in the neighborhood. My brother, sister and I all play with the kids up the street, who are close enough in ages though I am the youngest. They have some of the Marx Johnny West action figures, including Johnny, Jane, Geronimo, the covered wagon, the camping gear, and more. Most significantly for me, they also have some of the Marx horses including Thunderbolt and Storm Cloud. On rare days when the weather isn't as favorable to play outside, we break out these play sets. The other kids can play with the people. Leave the horses to me. I can't get enough, and often suggest that we stay inside and play "Johnny West" instead even on nicer days, but I am nearly always outvoted.

Except for a few pony rides, I've hardly even seen a horse let alone ridden one. But already, the attraction is apparent.

Little girls love horses. That's nothing new. But otherwise I suppose I can be considered a tomboy. My mother stuffs me into cute dresses and outfits, like her own little dress-up doll, but I don't enjoy it. I much more enjoy scuffling in the sandy soil wearing t-shirts, shorts and sandals until darkness forces us inside. I am impervious to the heat, and have no fear of the reptiles and amphibious creatures that abound here in great numbers. I develop an affinity for alligators, and I squeal with delight every time I see one, which makes our trip to the Florida Keys quite shrill.

While walking by myself to school one day, I have an altercation with a boy. We decide to settle this like big kids would, and arrange to meet on the sidewalk on the way home from school to duke it out. We agree it is to be just the two of us, no spectators.

We meet as agreed. No one else is around in this quiet community, and we make sure no one is watching. I am taller than him, so I figure I have the advantage.

"Don't hit me in the face," I warn. "My parents will get really mad."

He lets me throw the first punch, and I slam my fist into his stomach. He doesn't block me, but I am disappointed that he doesn't react. Now it's his turn, and he delivers in kind; a gut-wrenching punch that makes me want to double over and throw up. However, I am determined not to show weakness, so I fight back the discomfort, standing as tall and steady as I can. But I don't want to be hit again, so in a voice that struggles not to betray the success of his blow, I suggest we end it in a draw. He agrees and we each go home. I don't tell anyone about it for fear of getting into trouble. Years later, I realize that he probably was affected by my punch in the same way I was affected by his, and he was just as good at hiding it.

Chapter Four
Third of Three

"Have you seen that first grader with the messed up face?" a kid asks my brother.

"What about her?" Brian replies, bristling. "That's my sister." He's ready for a fight, which he narrowly avoids.

I am unaware of the altercation. I seldom hear what the other kids are saying about me behind my back. But if it isn't nice, they'd better not say it around Brian.

The oldest of us three and the only boy, he takes on responsibility as ward for his two younger sisters, though as strong-willed and aloof as our sister Lynne is, I doubt she needs or wants his protection.

Though defending me through the loyalty of blood, this does not preclude him from the firm belief that I am incredibly spoiled. Some of this could be simply because I am the youngest. Parents tend to be more rigid with their first and more flexible with later children since things that mattered initially don't matter anymore. Add to that all my medical needs, the unwanted notice of other children due to my altered appearance and the attention I require for hospital stays and doctor visits. Perhaps my parents are so grateful I am alive I often get concessions which I am happy to take advantage of.

While I don't mind getting my brother in trouble and often consider it a victory when I succeed, there is one line that simply is not to be crossed.

"The only reason she gets to do that I and don't is because of her face," he proclaims one day in frustration.

This results in howls of protest from me. The subject of my face is taboo in our house unless we are discussing future surgeries, and Brian knows it. It is very rare that he brings it up, which makes it all the more shocking.

"Mom, Brian mentioned my face!"

My mother's reaction is stern and immediate. Whether his assessment is accurate or not is beside the point. This time there is no joy from getting him in trouble. Rather, our house is my one guaranteed safe haven and I do my part to protect it.

I tear the blue and green wrapping paper off my gift and squeal with joy. There in front of me is my first Breyer model horse! My sister Lynne looks disgusted.

"She only wanted one because I have one," she says glumly.

Her sour response fails to dim my delight. Her horse is named Lightning, so I name mine Thunder. We share a bedroom, so they stand together on the shelf.

If imitation is the sincerest form of flattery, Lynne should feel honored. But she doesn't. Rather, she feels that her ability to be independent and unique has been thwarted by having a little sister tagging along demanding her attention and wanting everything she has.

Lynne finds herself firmly implanted in the limbo of being the middle child.

To her, I am the pesky little sister who always bugs her and her friends. I just want to be included and to not be alone, and I can justify being there since it's my room too. She just wants me to go away.

During my Middle School years, the family across the street has horses, and I am enthralled. The couple has only one child, a daughter Lynne's age named Rachel, and she and Lynne become friends. When Rachel offers to give me riding lessons on her mother's black gelding, I jump at the chance. I'd ridden before, but never had any sort of instruction. Though I don't consider Rachel and I to be friends because the age difference of two years is prohibitive, our common interest brings us together on a casual and friendly level. I look up to her and admire her, wishing I could have what she has, and she kindly tolerates this horse-crazy neighbor kid who happens to be Lynne's little sister. It doesn't occur to me that my sister may be jealous, feeling that I've intruded on their friendship.

While Lynne initially exhibits an interest in horses, they never become the obsession for her that they are for me. When Lynne is at home, we often hear the mellow tones of her violin or the woofing honk of her French horn through her closed door. Lynne is the musician of the family, active in band and orchestra. It is here she can be unique, as none of the rest of us are as impassioned with playing an instrument.

Lynne would rather be off with her friends doing band stuff than home with the family. It's not that she doesn't like us. She'd just rather be off doing her own thing.

Chapter Five
My Place in the Herd

In the summer of 1974, around the time I am turning eight years old, we leave Florida behind and return home to Washington. I expect us to move back to our old neighborhood where I will still have friends, and everything will be like it was before. I am disappointed when we don't.

The area we move to is on the opposite side of Puget Sound from where we used to live. This means starting in a new school with a whole new group of people who haven't seen my face before, so yet again I have to integrate into a new "herd."

A horse herd has a hierarchical structure. True alphas are fair leaders, and as long as their authority is unchallenged they pretty much leave everyone else alone. They enjoy the companionship of non-troublesome underlings, even allowing them to share their food. Further down the pecking order, however, some horses don't know how to handle authority. When they find themselves in the middle of the pack they often bully those below them, biting or chasing them for no other reason than to assert their superiority. Sometimes a clever individual will avoid such harassment by sticking close to an alpha and carefully staying out of trouble. The result of this is when a bully comes near, the alpha will pin its ears and drive it away, thus offering its underling companion a form of protection.

I am one such individual. I gravitate immediately to the company of the adults-in-charge, endearing myself to them so that I am able to stand in their protective shadow. I do this not only for protection, but also because it is from adults I get the most positive attention. Being a "favorite" or a teacher's pet makes me feel special. I like to feel special; I *need* to feel special. The uniqueness of my face is what initially garners extra attention from adult leaders since I do sometimes need shielding from the potential brutality of my peers. What I don't fully grasp at the time is that it's the personality behind the face that allows such status to continue. I *am* special.

Some children are jealous of the attention I get and lash out.

A sharp jab from one of my classmates startles me awake.

"Quit snoring!" I hear a sharp whisper as I jolt upright.

"Dawn's asleep again!" I hear someone say.

"I'm sorry," I express hoarsely, frustrated and embarrassed. I look around to see who's noticed. This time it's the whole class. I want to shrink into my chair.

I had struggled to stay awake but my eyelids were just too heavy. I snore loudly and am by necessity a mouth breather, which serves to both amuse and annoy my classmates.

"It's OK," the teacher replies. "Leave her alone. She can't help it."

"That's not fair," one boy proclaims. "We should all be able to sleep in class!"

Our teacher takes him to the nearby multipurpose room.

"Neither you nor I can possibly know what Dawn has been through," she explains to him gently. "She's a good student, she gets her work done, and she doesn't give me any trouble. Can you say the same?"

Likely my difficulty staying awake is caused by an obstruction of the airway which means I don't get the sleep I need at night. The study and diagnosis of sleep disorders such as apnea are in their infant stages and that connection is never officially made.

I can't stand in the shadow of the "alpha" figures constantly. There are times I am without protection, and at those times I am not immune from being bullied.

He lies in wait for me after school, like a stalker waits for a celebrity. Not an alpha, but rather someone who needs to feel superior.

"Hey, Face!" he matches me step for step. I try to ignore him. I put my head down and keep walking, a little quicker. The flight instinct is taking over and I aim for the security of a crowd. The predator will be less able to pick me off if I am in a group.

"How'd you get to be so ugly?" Every day, similar taunts.

"Why can't you just leave me alone?" I finally respond, the higher pitch of my voice betraying my distress.

"Because I can't stand being without you!"

I'm not physically afraid of him, but his verbal blows cut deeply and the nearly daily assault is taking its toll on my psyche. The periodic child's stare, a contorted facial expression, or an occasional taunt leaves its welt but is quickly forgotten. However I am not used to such blatant, persistent and deliberately cruel mockery.

I escape to the bus, landing heavily in the seat, relieved to be free of him for now but weighed down by his torment.

The school authorities are somehow alerted to his behavior and both sets of parents become involved. The issue is resolved and the teasing stops. Just as well for my tormenter, as my brother Brian had caught wind of it and he and his best friend were about to come over from the high school and pound on him.

Soon I would forget all about this. Perhaps I repress the memories, or perhaps while painful at the time, the situation isn't traumatic enough to make a lasting impression. Either way, I am able to put it behind me and move on.

Yet despite having been on the receiving end myself, I am not immune from being caught up in the bullying mentality.

Bert's family is poor. He and his siblings often come to school dirty and disheveled, and probably hungry. He is quiet and polite, and an average student. He doesn't seem to have many friends.

Some of the other children actively taunt him, while other times they make a point of avoiding him. I see them play keep-away with his things. I feel badly for him, but I am powerless to interfere. A part of me is grateful that it is him and not me and I feel guilty for having such feelings.

One day, Bert is walking alone down the hallway toward an exit. Today the game is to deliberately avoid anything he touches, spinning away from him as if he has a contagious disease.

"Look out! Here comes Dirty Berty!" one shouts. The others scatter away. There is no safe haven for him. No herd to meld into.

He approaches the door, trying to ignore them, but his face belies hurt and frustration. He just wants to get away. I am by the door along with a few others. He presses the metal bar and pushes the door open. The other kids scurry away. Struck by a sudden lemming-like compulsion, I spin away from Bert in the same mocking act of avoidance as the others. I stop dead in my tracks, instantly remorseful, mortified by my own action. This is not me. I may not be an alpha, but nor am I a bully. He meets my eyes as he slumps out of the building. I see pain reflected there. Betrayal; *Et tu?* A Brutus to his Cesar. I stare after him with guilt and shame.

I relate better to adults. The ones I interact with frequently, such as doctors, nurses, church leaders and teachers, treat me with respect. I long for adulthood, figuring that when I am an adult among adults, my face won't matter anymore.

I have a hard time relating to other eight-year-olds, and it seems to me that they have a hard time relating to me. Many of them are friendly in the way they interact with me, but very few are what I would consider friends. I don't hang out with them on the playground and they don't invite me over to play.

"Friend" is a conservative term for me. Since I am often not invited to birthdays and slumber parties, I have few casual friends. So when I call someone a friend, it is with great meaning.

I manage to find a friend in a quiet girl whom I am seated next to in class. Her name is Cora, and she doesn't seem to have many other friends either, which suits me fine because we can spend a lot of time together. Soon enough, we become best friends. However, when she does spend time with one of her other friends, I become possessively jealous. *What if she likes her other friend more than me? What if she decides to spend more time with her instead?* She is my only true friend, and without her I have no one. Suddenly my world seems terrifyingly lonely.

By the fall of '76, my upcoming surgeries will be less about stabilization and more about reconstruction and I can hardly wait. I try to visualize what my face would have looked like had all this not happened to me. I believe that these upcoming surgeries will fix my face and make it look like it should have been.

I don't even consider that if my face is "fixed," I might lose all this special status that I enjoy so much.

Chapter Six
Reconstruction

Destruction precedes construction. First they tore it all down. Then they laid a foundation for a future building site. Enough time has passed that the foundation has cracked a bit and needs some minor repair, but the construction workers had no choice but to wait. Build too soon and the stresses from growth rip it all asunder.

I am 10 years old now, and apparently this is the ideal age at which to begin reconstruction. I am old enough that my basic bone structure won't change significantly yet young enough to regenerate what can be regenerated and heal physical scars to the optimum.

There is much preparation to be done during the time preceding my first major surgery in eight years. I am just entering the fifth grade. My unsuspecting mind views the prospect of reconstruction as intriguing and interesting. I believe, despite the doctors telling me that this is the beginning of what could be many stages, that I will emerge with a symmetrical face. That very soon I will no longer be stared at or treated like an anomaly. I am looking forward to this.

The plan is for the surgeons to remove ribs and use them to reconstruct the bone structure of my jaw. Blueprints are drawn up and plans are made. The doctors need a look inside to see how my mandible remnant has grown and shifted and to assess jaw position relative to alignment.

I am planted in the chair of a panoramic x-ray machine, the design of which was undoubtedly borrowed from the

Inquisition. This dinosaur has a mouth piece intended for me to bite on. Since my upper and lower jaw are out of alignment, biting down is generally a challenge, so I am provided a plastic peg which swivels into place to rest my teeth against. A head piece swings down. The technician's wrist works feverishly turning knobs to make the fit small enough for a child. Pegs are stuck in my ears in order to steady my head and they jab uncomfortably at sensitive tissue. A heavy lead apron is placed over me. It covers my slight body almost completely, pinning me to the chair.

"Hold still for just a few moments!" the technician tells me as he vacates the room.

Under the weight of the apron, I can't move if I want to. I try not to allow my face to twitch as I wait a small eternity. The machine roars to life with a grind, a buzz and a whir. My ears hurt and I press against the mouth piece. An arm with a cylinder containing the film circles noisily in front of my face, slow and methodical. I follow its orbit with my eyes, willing it to hurry. When it finally settles to a halt, the technician returns, releases my head-lock, and excavates me from the apron. He pulls the panoramic film from the cylinder so he can develop it. I am returned to the waiting room where I fidget impatiently in the presence of my mother, but only after the film is developed and looks OK am I free to go.

I have no comprehension of what this is all for. I go where they point me and do what they tell me to do. It's all part of the process and I don't question it.

The pre-operative report refers to my situation as "post removal of facial teratoma with residual facial defect." So my deformity is a residue, like soap scum in the bath tub after a good soak. If only a good wiping down with the proper cleanser is all it would take to eradicate it.

On October 3, 1976, the night before my scheduled surgery, I am admitted to a university hospital.

After midnight, I am not allowed to eat. In the morning, an attendant comes for me with a gurney. Small and light, I roll easily onto it from my hospital bed. They swaddle me with blankets, but I shiver nonetheless with anticipation and nervousness. They roll me to the elevator and we all ride down to pre-op. Given my age, my mother is allowed to be with me. Double doors are pushed open before me as I enter a large room where I am parked against a wall.

I don't know how long I wait there, with nothing to do but ponder what might be coming next. Eventually the anesthesiologist, pushing a small table with ominous equipment, sits beside me on a rolling chair and introduces himself. He explains that he must insert an IV.

I do know enough to dislike needles, and I fight hard to keep my hand still for the prick which stings like fire. Gradually my hand numbs and he inserts the long hollow IV needle, praising me for my courage. My stomach growls uncontrollably. My high metabolism demands nourishment to produce more energy to burn, as my frail body has no such reserves. But in this environment, I am denied.

"Dawn, I'm going to give you something to help you relax. You'll feel a bit light-headed."

He squeezes a dose of sedation into the IV tube. It passes through me like a wave and the ceiling seems suddenly closer. The passing of time is more condensed, and soon I am wheeled away to the operating room. Before I leave my mother's side, she tells me that when I wake up it will be over.

The OR is cold and sterile. My surgeon, Dr. W, greets me in scrubs. They slide me from the soft gurney onto the hard cold slab of the operating table. I gaze in fascination and curiosity at the various apparatus with lights and beeps and noises. Though by today's standards it would be archaic, it is nonetheless awe-inspiring and effective.

"We're going to give you some oxygen, OK?"

I don't know why they turn it into a question, like it would matter if I said "no, it's not OK." I slur out some drugged response and they slip the clear mask over my mouth and nose. The oxygen assaults my senses. It's a terrible taste and smell, stale, dry and metallic. I wonder if it's possible for the metal canister it is being emitted from to flavor it.

"Breathe deep," I am instructed.

I comply, though I find it revolting.

I drift off, trying to take comfort in my mother's words. *When you awake it will be over.*

A surgical team extracts the fourth and sixth ribs from my left side. I've been assured that at my age they will grow back, an assurance that surprises me but I figure they should know.

A second surgical team of four, including Dr. W, then sets to work placing the grafts. Of the six surgeons participating, I only know two of them. I'm sure they've all been introduced as a matter of etiquette in the pre-op waiting area or in the OR, but their names and faces are unfamiliar to me. So I am mostly in the hands of strangers.

They slice through the existing scar tissue and free my right mandible, rotating it forward. An acrylic splint is placed between my teeth and my jaws are aligned in that fashion. In preparation for this procedure, I've had a full set of metal braces installed. The surgeons secure the jaw into position by wiring these braces together, top to bottom. On the left side of my face, they tighten things up, rotating and suturing loose soft tissue, muscle and scar tissue flaps to close the expanse left by missing bone so that the skin won't hang slack. A rib graft is trimmed to size then inserted. It is kept in place by threading wire through holes that have been drilled through the stub of the remaining mandible and through the newly inserted rib fragment and sewing the two together.

On my right side, a smaller rib fragment is sewn into place in a similar manner.

I am stitched up and the incisions dressed.

I am awakened in the operating room and brought to the intensive care unit in satisfactory condition. When I become conscious, however, I don't feel so satisfactory. Instead of it all being over, it is only just beginning.

Chapter Seven
Aftermath

I awaken to insistent hands pressing something firmly around my mouth and nose. Instinctively I try to move away from it, but I am only semi-conscious, drugged and weak. My face feels stiff and tight, and my jaws are unmistakably immobilized. I inhale but it is shallow as I become acutely aware that there is an intense pain as I try to draw in air. I am unable to take a deep breath. I am not in respiratory distress, as I seem to be able to get enough air, but my breathing is rapid, shallow and painful.

I look up pathetically in silent inquiry at the person who is putting a mask over my face. She moves it away momentarily.

"You've a partially collapsed lung," she explains. We need to pump air in to get it working again."

She places the mask with what looks to be a large black rubber balloon over my face. She holds it on firmly and compresses the bag slowly.

My eyes widen as the pain intensifies to the point of being all but unbearable. I don't fight back but I squirm uncontrollably in reaction to it. It doesn't help that the air they are forcing in smells and tastes like a tire.

"I know it hurts," she says. "But we have to do this. It's for your own good"

When she finishes the treatment, I am left aching. But that is not the end. It seems like every time I fall blissfully into painless slumber, I am awakened again by the black bag, pumping air deeply until my lungs feel they are about to explode. I envision my lungs as balloons which are stretched near to their limit, and dread the thought of one of them actually popping. They feel as if they might. The pain is excruciating. All night this goes on, despite my sleepy objections and pain-induced cries smothered in their wired prison.

The collapse was caused by a pocket of air or gas forming outside my lung, probably during the time my chest was opened for removal of the ribs. The treatment involves removing the external air pocket and then re-inflating the collapsed portion of the lung. Sounds simple enough, but it hurts like hell.

The treatments with the torturous black bag end by morning. That over with and feeling more awake, I am better able to assess my condition. My throat is raw and sore and I still have a feeding tube.

The nurse arrives with a cup of water and a syringe.

She looks me over.

"Oh, I guess you can't drink from a cup, can you dear?"

I shrug. She explains that many people with wired jaws are able to drink from a cup, but my barrier is too impervious. It doesn't help that I am unable to form any type of seal with my swollen lips and misshapen mouth, considering also the lack of muscle control on the left side of my face.

She uses the syringe to suck up some of the water.

"Here you go, dear. Can you do it or do you want me to help you?"

I reach for it, but my hesitation makes her continue.

"Just right in on the left side. There should be a place for it to fit there."

Awkwardly, I insert the nose of the syringe into the gap where several of my molars have been recently extracted. I gently compress the plunger and my mouth is filled with cool water. I sputter a bit as I try to control the liquid intake, regulate my airflow and coordinate swallowing. I am unable to breathe through my nose so I have to be careful not to drown myself. My throat is still sore from the surgery and its aftermath, so the cool liquid feels soothing going down. What amount of it that does go down, that is. Some of the water finds gaps in the wall of teeth and metal and oozes back out, across my helpless puffy chapped lips and down the front of my hospital gown.

The nurse wipes it up for me patiently.

"That'll take some practice," she remarks.

No kidding.

For lunch, I have a choice between vanilla and chocolate. White liquid or brown liquid delivered through the feeding tube with no possibility of tasting anything. I choose chocolate anyway. What kid wouldn't?

Where the IV is inserted, my hand is bruised and sore. The vein has shrunken to nothing and the needle is clearly defined through my discolored skin layers. This pain is more distracting to me than my bandaged swollen face, immobilized jaws or violated rib cage. It is my left hand, so I write hurried notes with my right hand begging for the removal of the IV.

"Not until you're eating and drinking," is the consistent reply.

The day after surgery, when I am settled into a regular hospital room, I am foisted out of bed on my doctor's orders. My legs want to buckle from weakness and my tender chest screams objections. I cannot speak clearly but I can make noise. Muffled cries mostly, but enough to get my opinion across. I am much happier suffering in a horizontal position rather than asking weak and undernourished muscles to perform.

They offer me no choice, but I am given help the first few times. One arm steadies me, another pushes the wheeled IV pole along; short distances at first until my stamina improves. Soon enough I am able to manage on my own.

On the way out the door for one such excursion, I pause at the mirror. I wish fleetingly that I were a vampire, whose image is unable to be reflected. Yet I study myself with curiosity and fascination. I look like I lost a fight. If I won I'd hate to see the other guy. My face is thick, distended and discolored. My left eye appears to have been punched; it is lined with black and olive bruising. My lips are fat, crusty and cracked since I cannot keep them moist and the frequent applications of salve don't seem to be enough. The left side of my face is puffy beneath the bandages. Dried blood, black and flaky, is encrusted around my ear and matted in my thick long hair, which is either pounded flat or sticking out oddly. I can see the last few x's of a line of black-threaded stitches protruding from beneath the bandage. I resemble Frankenstein more than any Disney princess. The skin around the incision is stained yellowish brown with iodine. I try not to be disappointed, but I cannot see past the swelling. I have to believe that things will improve with time and healing. It was made very clear that this is a first step. I shouldn't expect too much.

Wait until the swelling goes down, I remind myself. *That's when you'll start seeing a difference.*

The better I feel, the more bored I become. My increasingly frequent wanderings provide fleeting entertainment. I give myself a quick studying glance each time I pass the mirror, but nothing changes.

One drawback of having my surgery performed in a teaching hospital is that I become a specimen. Countless times, one of my doctors parades through a group of curious medical students and interns. He politely asks permission before entering, but who am I to refuse? Not that I can say much anyway with my mouth sealed shut. In they come, filling the room, staring intently with of course strictly professional curiosity as my case is briefly explained using words that are beyond my vocabulary. My case is, after all, quite unique. I feel awkward before this crowd of strangers who have come to stare at me intently, but at the same time I am flattered that my case is so interesting and I don't really mind being the center of attention.

The first fluid I am allowed to consume besides water is Ensure, which is high in calories. The consistency and color bear a strong resemblance to what has been dripping through my feeding tube, as does the choice between chocolate and vanilla. At least this I can taste, however.

When I am finally allowed food, the tray arrives with a selection of covered containers and several large sterile syringes still sealed in their plastic packaging. I eye the containers and my mouth waters with the anticipation of flavor. My mother uncovers the containers to reveal a warm clear broth which smells wonderful, a puree of some sort of vegetable, pureed apple sauce, a can of Ensure with an empty glass, and a lump of jell-o. We have a chuckle over that one. Apparently jell-o is considered part of a liquid diet, but it would be quite the challenge to suck that up a syringe. It hurts to laugh, but the pain is worth it.

Mother dips the nose of the syringe into the warm liquid and suctions it up. She hands it to me.

Eating has suddenly become an adventure. The more I eat, the sooner the IV can come out and free my suffering hand.

I remain relentless in pestering the doctors and nurses to remove the IV, through miming, gesturing, written messages, incomprehensible vocalizations, or any other means at my disposal. Finally, my liquid intake is considered sufficient, and I am freed from that painful tether. I can wander the halls more briskly now without the burden of pushing the IV pole around, or the arduous task of keeping tubing out from under my feet.

On October 9th, five days after surgery, I am discharged from the hospital with pain medication, dietary instructions, a huge stitched incision below what will become my left breast, a bruised hand, and a sore and swollen face. As far as I'm concerned, they can't push the wheelchair fast enough to get me out of there, though a whole new set of challenges await me at home.

Chapter Eight
Wired

Preparing meals for me becomes an art form. Water, milk, juice and broth become mixers as my mother and I try to liquefy foods enough to fit through a syringe without causing it to jam. The opportunities for experimentation presented by my special diet are fun and interesting, and most fruits and vegetables are not immune from a run though the blender. My food staples include thinned down mashed potatoes, baby meats blended with broth, pureed apple sauce, and yogurt shakes.

My first day back to school comes only days after my discharge. My face is still swollen and bruised and my eyes have dark circles under them. My classmates are curious, but at least at first don't attempt a lot of interaction. Maybe our teacher had a talk with them. My wired jaws keep me mostly quiet, and I carry around pen and paper with which to communicate.

By lunchtime I am exhausted, and I am relieved when Mother shows up with my meal. The school allows us to use an empty conference room so that I have privacy while eating since it would be embarrassing for me to eat in such a manner in front of my classmates. She arrives laden with thermoses and other sealed containers of liquid.

At first I enjoy the extra attention from my peers. They ask how I eat, and are amazed and jealous when I tell them I get to drink a lot of milkshakes. At lunchtime I am delighted when my mother either takes me home or we sequester to our private lunch room. But the novelty soon wears off. The concoctions that were at first so exciting for my mother and I to create have become bland and boring after being consumed day after day, week after week. I become increasingly jealous when I see other people eating solid food, and anything that smells good is pure torture.

Significantly, the communication barrier is wearing on me. I'd been told that many people with wired jaws are able to speak fairly intelligibly, but I am not one of those. I generally have a lot to say, so I find the lack of ability to verbally express myself frustrating. I feel gagged. I put monumental effort into my attempts to form words, to push my voice through the dense barrier, my lips struggling to form the correct shapes to aid with articulation.

"I'm sorry, I couldn't get that," I'm told. "Can you repeat that?"

Trying not to let my aggravation show, I make a second effort, this time more slowly. I feel like I'm yelling as I strive for more volume, projecting so hard my teeth hurt from the strain.

The responding look is pained and they shake their head, uncomprehending. "Sorry." It's all just muffled noises to their ears.

Exasperated, I madly scribble what I've been trying to say. But constantly writing out answers is time consuming and gives me writer's cramp. I crave questions that require either a yes or a no answer for which a nod or a shake will suffice.

I quickly give up on raising my hand in class even if I know the answer. I let the answer burn inside my head until someone else responds. Talking on the phone is out of the question. Playtime with Cora is more complicated since I can't engage in normal conversation.

There is one positive and unexpected consequence of this surgery, however. I am given a wider airway, likely due to forward movement of my jaw, which cures the apnea and allows me a better night's sleep. Thus ends my propensity to doze off in class.

Four weeks seem like four years. I am scheduled to have the wires cut just before Thanksgiving and I can hardly wait.

In the meantime, the swelling in my face gradually diminishes. The skin color returns to normal, and the soreness and bruising in my hand from the IV gradually fades away. I am amazed at how long the discoloration lasts. The stitches over my violated rib have been removed, leaving a long ugly red scar which curls up to my armpit. I can breathe and even laugh without feeling as if my ribcage is splintering.

I've also gained weight, which is my case is a positive thing. I had been very thin, due to a combination of high metabolism and fickle eating habits, but my appetite has increased and the liquid diet has provided a higher fat and calorie intake. I'm still small for my age, and proclaim that I want to be a jockey.

However, when I look in the mirror, I don't see much of a change from how I looked before the surgery. I quell my disappointment. *Give it time,* I tell myself. I don't allow myself to dwell on it. I'm too distracted by the inconvenience of my immobilized jaws, elated that soon this part of the ordeal will be coming to an end.

Seldom have I so looked forward to a doctor appointment, but I am all over this one. He has an x-ray taken first to be sure that everything has healed as expected.

I can't sit still in the waiting room. Dr. W is to do the honors, and by the time my mother and I are called in he has seen the x-rays and has determined that my jaws can be set free.

"I'll bet you're ready for this," Dr. W says amiably.

I nod enthusiastically.

"Just in time for turkey dinner," he adds.

"It would be difficult to put that in the blender," my mother comments.

"And being able to talk," I say. Weeks of practice and diminished facial swelling have enabled me to push some words through more comprehensibly.

"Oh, yeah, we all can't wait for that," says Mother with good natured sarcasm.

As I sit back in what is effectively a dental chair, he carefully positions me and then goes meticulously to work. A snip and a pull free one bond. The restraining wires must be carefully cut and unstrung without affecting the braces which need to remain intact. Another snip and tug, and another and another. He works slowly and meticulously. I lie still despite my impatience. I just want him to be done. His last effort is to remove the molded hard resin retainer from between my teeth, which has kept everything in a fixed position.

"That should do it," he says, sitting back. He gets up and washes his hands.

To my surprise, my lower jaw doesn't want to move at all. There is a slight gapping from the release of the restraining wires, and I draw air through it with a deep inhale. But I still feel immobilized. I expected everything to be back to normal again once the wires were cut so I am confused.

"I can hardly move," I say with effort. Free of the constraints, my muscles try to position my jaws as I would in normal speech, but they are too stiff and the effort too painful. At least my voice is significantly less muffled.

"It's going to be stiff," says the doctor, noting my reaction. "I'm going to show you some exercises to help stretch the muscles and get things working again."

He sits me up in the chair and holds up his hands.

"What you need to do is to hold your fingers like this," he says. He crosses his thumb and forefinger and moves them in a scissor-like fashion. He moves them to my mouth and gently applies pressure with the thumb on the upper teeth and forefinger on the lower. My jaw begrudgingly begins to open. It hurts, but at least it is moving.

"Now you try it," he says, drawing his hands out.

I insert my fingers as demonstrated and push. Self-inflicted, I have a much higher pain tolerance, but the jaw opens only so much and the resistance is too great. I push until I can't stand the pain any longer.

"You'll need to do this 4 or 5 times a day, about 10 repetitions each time," he advises. "Start with soft foods."

He sends me home with instructions and dietary recommendations, and I am to continue to wear the retainer now held in place with rubber bands instead of wires.

I do the exercises much more often than recommended. Despite the diet change, my stomach is no worse for wear. On Thanksgiving, I eat twice what everyone else does.

My family can't shut me up. I have a lot of stored up words that come flooding out.

Chapter Nine
When Wishes Are Horses

By age 11, I am aware that some people have only a passing attraction to horses, like my sister for example. I discover that many little girls who are so taken with them in childhood outgrow their interest. Some rekindle it years later, but many never do.

I will always love horses, I proclaim to myself. And somehow I know it to be true.

It is sometime in the fourth grade that my best friend Cora draws me into the world of model horse collecting. Aside from our original pair, my sister and I have acquired a scant grouping of Breyer model horses of maybe a dozen or so, but I haven't yet entertained the idea of being a serious collector.

As the car climbs up the long gravel driveway toward Cora's old white two storey farmhouse for the first of what would be many visits over a period of years, I gaze out enviously at the large fenced pastures on either side. My mind's eye sees the potential for fields full of horses, but alas there are none. Only chunky beef cattle, brown and black, grazing away. One or two look up as we pass but we are quickly ignored in favor of diminishing grass under cloven hooves.

Cora has horses, but not the kind found out in the field. Rather, she stables hers in the living room, under a cement slab that serves as the hearth for the fireplace insert. There must be at least 30, side by side in a colorful row, staring out at us.

I am transfixed. The colors, the shapes, the expressions… and there are so many! Breyer Animal Creations strives for proportion and scale, and uses talented sculptors to create the works from which their molds are constructed, so many of their models have a more realistic appearance than other toy horse statues. Some of these have seen better days with rubs in the paint and tape holding together broken legs despite the robust plastic they are molded from, but that is of little consequence. Never have I seen so many in one place. I am instantly awed and envious. I kneel down to have a closer look, and Cora is all too happy to show them off.

The model horses become our principal play toys. They all have names, and we invent whole new worlds and societies for them to live in. At first we include dolls and Barbie-type figures, but humans soon become vile creatures who only seek to disrupt the natural wild state of the horses. Eventually humans are written out of the script completely. After all, the horses have magical powers so they are able to get by quite adequately without opposable thumbs.

The herd grows. Each new purchase or gift is introduced as a new "herd member" at our next time of play. But we always fall back on our favorites, and they are worse for wear because of it. The model horses are alive to us. Our imaginations run rampant. Our equine society evolves and changes along with our increased awareness of the world around us. Politics and corruption eventually litter our story lines.

Indoors, outdoors, their world exists wherever we can carry them. In the yard, out in the fields, into the woods, along streams. We play for hours, impervious to cold or heat, daylight or darkness. At night we watch them in the dimness, waiting for them to start moving. They in turn watch over us with fixed expressions.

My horse statues are my imaginary friends with a physical form. Some children have soft plush teddy bears. I have cellulose acetate equines. They are my sentinels and my companions. Like a security blanket, I carry them to doctor appointments and to school. I set them up in front of the television to watch with me. Which ones I bring to the TV with me depends on which show is on. After all, they have favorites too.

My interest in the model horses transforms over time from play things to collectibles. I become more grateful that we played less with mine and more with Cora's, hence sparing mine the wear and tear and allowing more of my earlier pieces to remain in collectible condition.

We obsess on live horses as well. Cora imagines that she'll inherit the farm someday, and we plan to turn it into a grandiose horse facility. We will own a breeding pair of all the different horse breeds we can think of. Beautiful, elegant and exotic breeds such as Friesians, Andalusians, Lippizans and Paso Finos. We envision our adult selves riding gorgeous stallions with long flowing manes.

We tear obsessively through Walter Farley's The Black Stallion series and devour every horse story we can find. I take to reading breed books, which are generally dry and factual, but I devour the pictures and descriptions. It is in one such breed book that I first read about the Icelandic horse.

That looks exotic, I think to myself. *I'll probably never see one, let alone ride one. But they do look like fun.* Icelandic horses never come up in our conversations and long term plans.

My own dreams of owning a horse in my youth never come to fruition, even though my family has property. Disappointed about not having a horse of my own, I instead go around the neighborhood and ask people if I can ride their horses. I am occasionally successful, but more often then not owners don't want to take the risk that I might get hurt on their horse. Their concern baffles me.

When Cora's parents purchase a horse for her, I am elated, as I figure I'll finally have a chance to ride a lot more often.

Poco is a tall, sturdy horse, easy to catch and tolerant of our amateur status. We are fearless and indestructible at this age. With one horse and two of us, we take turns or ride double. We just get on and we go. No lessons, no helmet, no heeled shoes, no clue. It feels good up there, lumbering around on this giant equine. All I know about riding is

to get on and do it. You kick to go, move your hand side to side to steer, and pull back to slow down or stop. It will be a few years yet before I connect with my sister's friend Rachel and take lessons for the first time, and years after that before I truly learn how to ride.

We never seem to ride as much as I'd like to. A professor once told me that the definition of *to have* is "to cease to desire," which he accredited to Ambrose Bierce's *The Devil's Dictionary*. He must have been paraphrasing. Regardless of its origin, the phrase seems to ring true, as once the newness of having a horse wears off, Cora doesn't seem all that interested in riding anymore. I express my disappointment, but since he is hers and not mine, I have little say.

Having a live horse in the picture doesn't take away from our adventures with the model horses. It just gives us more options.

While a good horse in many respects, Poco nonetheless demonstrates a destructive, dangerous and expensive habit of uprooting small trees and breaking posts the size of telephone poles when it's time to have shoes put on, so he is eventually sold. He is soon replaced by two others, so at least on the seemingly rare occasions when we do ride, we can ride together.

Chapter Ten
Setbacks

By the time I get to middle school, I've been with pretty much the same kids for three years. I have more casual acquaintances, but there are still not many whom I consider friends, especially since I use the term sparingly. A part of me believes I want to be popular and have lots of friends because that would signify acceptance. However, the reality I haven't admitted to myself yet is that I actually prefer having a couple of intimate friends rather than spreading my time and attention too thin. Besides, I can be intense and tend to express myself rather bluntly. But I don't think about such things as being a turn-off for potential friends. In fact, I don't think about such things much at all.

Seeking a way to be more involved and to put my organizational talents to use, I decide to run for secretary in the student body election. I believe I have a chance of becoming elected, or else I would not be running. I'm not in it for the learning process. I'm in it to win. But it seems to be a popular position seeing as I have four competitors.

I may not have many friends, but I have enough to get nominated. After all, it only takes one. This is my first brush with politics. I may not be popular, but to my knowledge I am not disliked. I have the advantage of being recognizable, and I am definitely qualified.

I draw up and hang posters and give my campaign speech at the student assembly in an effort to get my name and face associated with the office I am running for. I emphasize my strengths: I am organized, a hard worker and a good writer.

Election day rolls around and the ballots are cast. When the votes are tallied, all the candidates are called into the office. We get to find out the results first so there are no surprises, thus sparing the losers public displays of disappointment.

I am one of the losers.

It was probably very close, my ego declares.

"Can I see the vote count?" I ask.

"We don't give out that information," the office staff person tells me.

I bear the news with head held high, despite the bitter wave of disappointment. The victor is someone I know and like. While I did not perceive her as being especially popular, she was obviously more popular than I.

The reality might be that I had no chance and lost by a landslide. I may have been lucky to get more votes than can be counted on my fingers. But my ego shields me from that eventuality. That's what egos are for.

Murray, a classmate who eventually becomes a close friend, disagrees.

"Of course you had a chance to win," he declares. "But in a contest between popularity and competence, and how else can you expect a bunch of pre-teens to vote?"

"How can we say that the person who won isn't also competent?" I reply. "For that matter, I didn't think she was all that popular."

I am recognizable, outgoing and vocal. But there is a difference between having everyone know who you are and being popular.

"You'd have stood a much better chance had it not been a secret ballot," Murray reasons. "Who would dare vote against poor Dawn in a public vote?"

I can only stare at him in amazement. I certainly do not perceive that my classmates pity me. I weigh his words over time.

No, I conclude. *I don't believe that to be the case.*

It hardly matters. The end result is that I not only lose the election, but I lose a lot of confidence as well. I naively believed that my qualifications and drive would earn me the acceptance of my peers and therefore the victory. I was wrong. I do not run for any more school offices after this. I don't handle losing very well, so I choose not to risk further humiliation and defeat.

To make matters worse, I am reaching an age where physical attraction is becoming more significant. Hormones are kicking in. I certainly lack the face that launches a thousand ships. I'm not sure mine even warrants a dinghy. I have neither a Siren's song to lure suitors or Medusa's stare to turn them to stone, and there are definitely times I wish I could do one or the other. Boys I am attracted to have no interest in me except as a friend, if even that.

Periodically, a guy will elbow another guy in his group, point at me and proclaim loudly "Hey, there goes your girlfriend!" He and his lackeys then have a good laugh at their friend's expense, as if he is so witty and original. I assure you, he is neither. I either do my best to completely ignore the comment, or else I send them a look made up of equal parts shock, hurt and anger, then walk hastily on, wounded but trying not to dwell on it. *Who says I'd want to be his girlfriend anyway? He's not my type.*

But the distressing reality is that to my pubescent peers I am simply unattractive, and my appearance is not enhanced whatsoever by being back in braces.

By September of 1978, it is apparent that my jaws have slipped out of alignment, so my doctor suggests more surgery. This has been anticipated so is not a surprise to me or my parents. It will be similar to the previous surgery in that another rib graft will be transplanted into my cheek. This one will be added onto the existing transplants to regain alignment and further reconstruct the jaw. I don't expect any magical enhancements for this one. This is another preparatory step toward what I hope will be significant changes later on.

The procedure is scheduled for June 25th, 1979, shortly after school lets out for the summer. I've just completed 7th grade.

As before, I look forward to this surgery. There still exists the notion that someday I will look normal, but in the short term it offers a way I can be the center of attention. Each time, I manage to repress the pain and suffering associated with the process so that I have the outcome to look forward to. However, I do not relish having my jaws wired shut again for either the bland boring menu or the nightmare of trying to communicate. At least I won't be in school this time.

I am admitted the night before, enduring the usual unrest associated with a hospital room that is constantly changing temperature, an insufficient hospital garment, the frequent awakenings caused by nerves and anticipation, late night blood draws, and the early morning arrival of the orderly to cart me away on a cold thin gurney to pre-op. Once again I shiver uncontrollably, which no heated blanket can remedy.

The needle, then the IV insertion; I've suffered it all before and it doesn't get any easier with practice.

I am awake as they wheel me into OR, where I am greeted by Dr. W and the usual entourage of surgeons, assistants and the anesthesiologist. I hear the familiar ping of equipment and the clink of tools being set out; the recognizable sounds of preparation. Soon enough, I blissfully slip away.

Under the influence of anesthesia, I am completely unaware of the passage of time. I do not dream. My consciousness drifts, and what seems like seconds later I am waking up. But of course time has passed and as my brain fights the fog and my eyes reluctantly open, I become acutely aware of the results of what my body has experienced in my mental absence. Depending on the procedure and the drugs, the sensation I awaken to is not always pain. Sometimes it is tightness, sometimes a lack of control over a certain portion of my body, sometimes discomfort.

This time I become almost instantly aware of what didn't happen. My throat feels raw and swollen but not obstructed and my breath is labored and raspy. Most significantly, however, my lower jaw is slack. I ask my brain to send a signal to my jaw. It moves!

It's not supposed to do that, I conclude groggily.

"Dawn." A familiar voice penetrates the haze.

I try to locate the source.

"Dawn, it's Dr. W."

Somehow speaking doesn't seem like a good idea.

"We had to abort the procedure," he explains. "We couldn't get the breathing tube in."

I am not sure whether to feel disappointment or relief.

"You have a lot of swelling," he continues. "We've decided that it would be best to postpone."

Disappointment wins. I'm here. I have been ready for this to be done and over with. Now I'm going to have to go through all this again.

I remain in the hospital for another day, during which I primarily sleep. The swelling is significant and my throat is sore and I am so hoarse my voice is barely audible. The next day I am breathing better and the swelling has decreased so I am sent home with an oral pain medication.

I am told I have a very difficult airway due to anatomical distortions. According to Dr. W, only about 1% of people in the anesthesia profession are skilled enough to successfully manage it. This particular hospital is fortunate to have such a gifted professional on staff. Unfortunately for us and unbeknownst to Dr. W when he scheduled my procedure, this particular professional is out of town. Another anesthesiologist tried unsuccessfully for well over an hour before the swelling in my throat got so bad that continued attempts were impractical. No wonder my throat is so sore. I am relieved I wasn't awake for it.

The plan is to reschedule for another hospital where there is more anesthetic expertise. In the meantime, I am left with pain and no gain and the certain knowledge that I have more suffering ahead of me. On the bright side, I get to enjoy my summer a bit more.

Chapter Eleven
Here There Be Dragons

My world can be lonely and painful, so I spend time in other worlds instead. My friend Cora and I invent a universe in which our model horses come alive. My mother takes me through the wardrobe, reading me the entire Chronicles of Narnia. So captivated am I that I later make the journey on my own. I spend time as a dragonrider on Pern, I travel Middle Earth with Bilbo and Frodo, and am enchanted by the magical powers of Aslan, Merlin and Gandalf.

Inspired by being read to and then in turn by reading, I've been writing stories since grade school.

"I've written another play. It's a Christmas play. Can we perform it for the class?" I ask my fifth grade teacher. She is happy to nurture my creativity.

I recruit my few friends and the teacher handpicks responsible classmates to fill out my cast. We are allowed to rehearse unattended in the multipurpose room during class time. It doesn't occur to me that there is anything unusual about that. We have a task to do and we do it, like the responsible little ten-year-olds we are. We make our costumes from construction paper, and our sets are tables and chairs which a child's imagination can mold into any object in any location.

We perform not only for our own class but for the other classes as well. I am very nervous, but excited that something I've orchestrated gets a public showing. I am not only writer and director, but I take on a primary acting role as well. For this Christmas play, I am the chief reindeer, crowned in paper antlers. Hidden off to one side, I carefully wait for my cue, then interrupt the conversation of two other characters with loud, raucous snoring. This simple yet effective comic device gets the desired result: the audience laughs. However, I cannot stop myself from laughing with them, making it hard to continue my lines. But it's worth it. Intentionally or not, I am playing up one of the very things I am known for- falling asleep in class and snoring. Yet they are not laughing at me. They are laughing because I want them to.

Since this unstructured masterpiece doesn't have a planned conclusion, the teachers bring it to an end when the improvisation falls flat, the plot or the actors start to wander aimlessly, and the class runs out of time.

I generate several of these, and my imaginative efforts land me a spot in the Enrichment Language Arts program. This program nurtures writing talent, teaching ways for the student to enhance creative and descriptive skills. Here, I explore different writing styles including prose and poetry. I am considered "gifted," a label I enjoy because it means I am better at something than many other kids my age. I flourish in this program. Most of my writings are fantasy unless a specific project dictates something else. It is easier to make up my own world than to study and research the one I live in.

There's a foul stench of dampness, rotten meat and decay in the air as I glide silently along the rock-hewn wall, an odor worse than that of my companions. My belongings, including a pack, a bow and a sword, are strapped tight against my person so as not to clank and rattle, and I have a dagger ready in my nimble hand. Close combat is not my forte. I am much more adept at prying locks and finding and disabling traps. I've been known for a little, "slight of hand" work as well, lining my pockets with a few extra gold pieces. Snug leather armor protects me from the roughness of the wall I am hugging and Elven eyes allow me to see without a lantern or torch. I hear gruff voices ahead of me which cause me to pause, holding my breath as I listen intently. I do not understand the words but I recognize the language. The tenor seems unalarmed so I crouch low and inch forward. I have to be sure... The faint light flickering ahead tells me they'll be just around this corner. I reach the edge of the room, staying just out of the light, and my suspicions are confirmed. Orcs! That explains the rotting meat smell. There are about half a dozen, hide armor and simple weapons. They'll be no match for us. I retreat slowly. I have to report this to the others. I make it about 20 feet when suddenly part of the load I am carrying shifts unexpectedly causing my long sword to smack the wall with an audible clang. I hear the voices behind me change pitch and the unmistakable clamor of mobilization. My stealthy retreat blown and facing certain slaughter if they catch me, there is only one option: RUN! "ORCS!" I scream as I vault toward my party. I am lighter and faster than they are. I should make it back to my group ahead of them, where my companions will be ready to engage. At least that is how I hope it will play out...

I am 12 years old, sitting around a table with my friend Darren and his two younger brothers playing Dungeons and Dragons (D&D). The attributes of our characters are spelled out on sheets before us, obscured slightly by cookie crumbs and soda can rings. Our characters are represented by painted metal figures, trekking through the halls and rooms of a dungeon module mapped out on large scale graph paper. Darren is our dungeon master, enlightening us of each new discovery, revealing the map as we go and introducing us to each adversary.

The two characters I play represent a chance to be someone else for awhile. I prefer my characters to be non-human because it makes them more exotic and often gives them special abilities. I enjoy the opportunity to escape every day reality yet apply tactics and make choices that could mean life or death for my character. It is a game of imagination and visualization, aided by drawings, illustrations and figures on the table. Of course the element of chance is mixed in, as success or failure is often determined by the roll of a die. When Ayron, my Elven thief in the previous narrative, fails to make good his stealthy escape, it is because I'd rolled below the number he needed to succeed with his "sneak" ability.

Role playing at its best allows the player to think and act as his or her character would, but I'm not quite into it that deeply. But I enjoy the escape, the intimacy, and the humor of our gaming sessions, always looking forward to them and sorry when our time is up. When the natural progression of childhood ends our sessions for good, it will be 15 years before I take up role playing games again.

While I am not the sort to turn the TV on and sit for hours watching nothing unless I am home sick from school, I do have my favorite shows and I tend to be obsessed with them and their main characters. My favorite show for its first several seasons is *Fantasy Island*, and I turn obsession turns to inspiration.

In the fall of '79 I craft my first Fantasy Island script. I use the term "script" loosely because I know nothing at this time about screenplay format. I write the entire project in prose. The first draft is in pencil, but later I bang it out on a manual typewriter using the sophisticated two-finger typing technique.

It is my longest writing to date, and is truly a labor of love. There is no school assignment attached to it, nor is it associated with anything I am doing for the Enrichment Language Arts program. I have an idea and I begin to write. The story forms as it hits the page, and I don't stop until it winds its way to an unplanned but logical conclusion. I dream of having my story produced on the show and getting to visit the set and meet the actors. I have no concept of how to obtain this unrealistic goal.

However, once written, I take it to my Enrichment Language Arts instructor to show it off.

To say she is impressed by it is an understatement. She in turn hands it off to a friend of hers, an actress who is currently one of the co-hosts of a morning TV show in Seattle. She still has Hollywood connections, and unbeknownst to me she passes my manuscript off to a friend of hers.

Not long after, I am surprised to receive a package in the mail from producer/writer Allan Burns. He has sent me a letter commenting on my story, as well as a couple of the scripts he has written. One is the Emmy-award-winning script for *Mary Tyler Moore*, "The Last Show," and the other is an Emmy nominated script from *Lou Grant*. He explains that these should help me learn the screenplay format. Though he says my dialogue is a bit stilted, he thinks the story-telling is impressive and compliments me for my ability to jump back and forth between two completely separate storylines without confusing or losing the reader. He says this is very difficult to do and I handle it quite well. I am thrilled.

What incredible inspiration for a 13 year old. As far as I am concerned, I am on my way to Hollywood. My career goal becomes quite clearly *Screenwriter*. I respond to Mr. Burns' letter and begin studiously learning the teleplay format.

Chapter Twelve
The Bitter Suffering of Success

Not long after I begin my freshman year in high school, my doctors decide it is time for "take two" on the procedure that had been aborted the previous year.

The plan is the same as before: reconstruction of the jaw using rib grafts and shifting the left side forward and more into alignment. Lacking computerized visual imaging, the doctors simulate the desired results of the surgery on a plaster model. They take measurements and manufacture an acrylic index, or splint, which is shaped to fit a section of teeth on the upper jaw and a corresponding section of teeth on the lower jaw. During surgery, this splint becomes the guide for orienting the jaw segments. When my jaw is properly aligned, my teeth will fit neatly into the splint, after which time they will wire my jaws in place. This of course means another month of eating via a syringe, which I am *not* looking forward to.

In order to avoid a repeat of the previous intubation fiasco, a specialist has been called in. On October 16, 1980, I am wheeled into the OR and lifted to a sitting position. They've pumped a sedative through the IV and I am very groggy, but the anesthesiologist requires that I be awake for what he must do.

"Dawn," Dr. W addresses me. "Dr. Michaels is going to insert the breathing tube now."

Dr. Michaels approaches me.

"I need you to open wide," he says. He holds up a small

spray bottle. "I'm going to spray this on your throat to make it numb. You need to keep your tongue down and out of the way."

I open my mouth as best I can. He holds up the bottle and sprays its liquid contents as deeply toward the back of my throat as he can.

I gag, and gag again, shaking my head violently. It is not merely the contact of a foreign substance on tender tissues of my mouth and throat. This has got to be the foulest tasting concoction I've ever experienced and my body rejects it spasmodically. I am not groggy enough.

He comes at me with it again and I shake my head violently. He looks helplessly to Dr. W, who takes my hand firmly and speaks to me gently.

"I know it's terrible stuff, but we need to do this or else we can't proceed. Try and lie still."

Wild-eyed but determined to following instructions, I allow another application and involuntarily gag again. But it's starting to have the desired effect. My taste buds are still assaulted by the bitterness and my throat feels like it is sealing up. I gulp breaths because the deadening of the nerves in the throat fool my brain into thinking that my breathing is impeded. This is not the case, but I can no longer feel the air moving through my mouth and down into my lungs and it is disconcerting and scary.

"Now just try to relax. We're going to insert the tube."

I do my best to lie still, but relaxing is not an option.

"Now take deep breaths," he instructs.

I do my best to take what I think are long deep breaths, going through the motions by memory because I can no longer go by feel.

The anesthesiologist begins to insert the tube. I feel it probing and stabbing my throat wall and I resist turning my head away and try desperately to control the gagging and choking.

"Keep breathing," he says.

My breathing is his guide. He listens to the movement of the air, which tells him where to direct the tube.

The numbness of the noxious spray only penetrates so far, and the sensation of rubber tubing on raw unprotected membranes is indescribable. It is akin to touching an area in which all the skin has been peeled back and the nerve endings exposed. It takes an agonizing 15-20 seconds to complete the insertion. The capable hands of this anesthesiologist perform a successful blind intubation on the first attempt and I am blissfully sent to unconsciousness.

To me those seconds are an eternity which has emblazoned itself into my memory. I am able to taste and reflexively respond to that noxious gagging spray for approximately 15 years following its application.

No matter how unpleasant this experience, the alternative would have been a tracheostomy which I am glad to have dodged. That is one scar I prefer not to have reopened.

Since they've already taken ribs from the right side, this time the ribs will be extracted from the left. Good thing I have so many of them. Now I will have matching scars.

The surgeons use the rib extractions to build up the healthier right side of my face. On my left side, they find that the previous graft has healed firmly into place. However, the goal is to move the jaw forward, so the old anchor wires from the previous surgery are cut and removed and the bone or semblance of bone along with any tissue that might inhibit such movement is dissected. This, however, does not leave my jaw free-floating, which needs to happen in order for them to proceed. They then work through my mouth, using considerable force to wrest the mandible free from any restraining soft tissue. Now they are able to bring the jaw forward and rotate it into position. The carefully crafted acrylic splint is inserted and the jaws are wired into place using my braces. In an effort to replace my missing cheek bone and add some contour, they sandwich two rib pieces together to construct a ledge in the appropriate position.

Since they don't yet have the option of using bone plates and bone screws, which give more latitude and stabilize the area during healing, everything needs to be held together by wires. To this day, I cannot have an MRI on my face and head due to interference by the amount of metal present. It's a wonder I don't set off metal detectors!

I wake up in post-op violently nauseous from the anesthesia. My empty stomach heaves saliva and blood, trapped by the wall of teeth sewn together by wire. The taste of blood, vomit and stomach acid is dreadful. I turn to rid my mouth of the revolting liquid but there is no easy exit. What dribbles free is flecked with black specks, which I can only guess is dried blood. What cannot escape, which is most of it, must be suctioned out. Swallowing is not a preferable option.

This didn't happen last time, my tortured brain moans as I suffer another wave, confused that my body should choose such an adverse reaction to the anesthesia this time around.

Each heave strains my newly sealed jaws until I feel like all my teeth might separate from my gums. The muscle convulsions tear at the fresh incision where my ribs have been newly harvested. My frustrated sobbing only compounds unwanted movement in my abdomen.

"You poor thing," the attending nurse says kindly. "And with your jaws wired, too."

She does the best she can to clear my mouth before the next involuntary effort adds to it.

After another miserable eternity, and probably with the help of medication, the nausea subsides.

Meanwhile, someone decides that I need to have blood drawn every 10 minutes. Ok, it was probably every hour but it might as well have been every 10 minutes. I have good veins, or so I've been told by nearly every medical professional who has ever drawn my blood. After about the fifth time, however, those veins dive into the innermost recesses of my arm. I scream and cry through wired jaws for the orderly taking blood to STOP after about the fourth unsuccessful jab, but he is unrelenting.

Soon even this misery also passes into memory and the torture repressed. The hospital staff have me up and moving as quickly as possible and I am discharged three days after my surgery.

Chapter Thirteen
Distractions and Motivations

While other freshman are adjusting to the rigors of high school life, I'm working twice as hard to catch up on class work and not fall further behind as I juggle doctor appointments and continue the arduous task of trying to heal.

Having one's jaws wired the second time is not nearly as intriguing as the initial experience. My mother and I are dry on ideas for new menu items to try and the same old stuff seems bland and boring. Meals are once more major events, though this time around I am more likely to pack my lunch to school and find a private place where I can manage on my own. Communication yet again becomes complicated and frustrating.

To add to my stress, I've come to the sudden realization that if I want to get into college I'll need to improve my grade point average. In middle school I was an average performer because I didn't apply myself, but high school is a chance at a fresh start so I am determined to get the best grades I can.

I watch the swelling go down and my face take on a disappointingly familiar shape. I didn't expect miracles or dramatic improvements this time around, but for all the suffering something notable would have been nice. Even the built-up cheek bone doesn't offer anything that I can point to and say *hey, I can see the difference!* But the internal structure is changing, lining up my jaws and improving my bite. At least the braces are giving me straight teeth.

Though I don't realize it at the time, I am about to enter a two and a half year hiatus from surgical procedures, putting on hold my quest for the perfect face. I still believe improvements are achievable, but I'm OK with waiting. Though my brain is expert at repressing the memories of pain and inconvenience associated with surgery, it still takes some time for that repression to kick in. The scars are all too fresh, and besides, I need to concentrate on my studies.

As *Fantasy Island* did before, the show that motivates me creatively is *The Greatest American Hero*. I am enfatuated not with the cute young blonde hero with the super suit he doesn't know how to use, but rather his gruff sarcastic sidekick Bill Maxwell. By this time, thanks to the scripts sent to me by Allan Burns and to private tutoring, I know how to write a teleplay in the correct format. I create two original screenplays for the show, my head once again full of dreams of having my stories produced and therefore meeting the cast. With this goal in mind, I send a letter to Stephen J. Cannell, producer of the series, and eagerly await a reply.

What I get is a black and white glossy of the three main characters and a bumper sticker. While cool and nice to have, my heart sinks. In a letter to Allan Burns, I lament this response.

A few weeks later, I receive a personal letter from Mr. Cannell, apologizing that my original correspondence had been mixed in with the fan mail, encouraging me to keep writing, and offering to read my scripts as a sample of my work even though the show has been canceled. I am elated. But I am young and inexperienced. After some confusion about where to send the scripts (apparently Stephen J. Cannell Productions is in the midst of moving to a new building), I receive what I perceive as a curt letter from Mr. Cannell's secretary and a two-page release form. The letter in reality is straightforward and non-threatening, but at age 16 I find it intimidating and never send the manuscripts. I often wonder how mailing those might have changed the path of my life.

"You should go see Mr. Grayson," a teacher advises upon learning of my propensity for writing screenplays.

Being somewhat shy about introducing myself to a stranger, I put off this meeting for awhile. Despite getting along with adults more easily than I do my peers, I still look upon adults as authority figures. Even as I evolve as a free-thinking human being, the notion of adults as equals hasn't quite germinated in the fertile soil of my developing brain.

Mr. Grayson is the sole staff occupant of the former music building, a new construct having taken over this purpose several years prior. It is his kingdom. One day after school I nervously approach this fortress with its double glass doors. The entry is adorned with old movie posters, mostly for films unfamiliar to me. There are some student projects hanging on the wall, and a sign that boldly proclaims *Media Now*, which is one of his most popular courses. Once inside the building, I turn left and enter the classroom through yet another door. It is a large room with a high ceiling and a tiered floor that once accommodated the rows of students playing musical instruments.

Standing near a podium at the front of the room, gathering up the day's materials, is a raven haired man with a dark mustache, each betraying the beginnings of the graying process. His back is slightly hunched but he nonetheless stands erect. He greets me with bright laughing dark eyes.

"How-doody," he says. "What can I do you for?"

"Mr. Grayson?"

"That would be me."

"I'm Dawn. I write screenplays and am interested in the movie and television industry and I was told to come talk to you."

Thus I introduce myself to my most motivating force in high school. Mr. David Grayson. Writer, teacher, and mentor.

I spend many hours after school with Mr. Grayson. He shares with me some of his writings, mostly in essay format, which he has since published in his own book. I start writing some of my own essays and share them with him.

Once an English teacher, he has branched out to teaching all forms of media, and maintains the only Speech class. I take his popular *Film Study* course, in which we primarily watch movies. I give him my *Greatest American Hero* scripts to read.

After reading my screenplays, he announces to the whole class that my stories are better than most of what he's seen on television. I am simultaneously proud and embarrassed.

I seek any excuse to spend time with him. I am totally taken with him and fall into a full-fledged high school crush. Whether this is healthy or not, it gives me focus. It motivates me to take on certain projects I might not otherwise have done, and to keep writing. For example, I win an award at the regional level for a political speech I had thrown together because Mr. Grayson was the faculty advisor. My success is likely due to my talent as a writer and ability to deliver it eloquently. Despite what I perceive to be an impaired voice, I do have a sense of timing and a flare for the dramatic. Or perhaps my victory was due to lack of competition.

He doesn't seem to mind me hanging around excessively. He puts me to work when he has it, gives me reading materials, and behaves perfectly toward me. We even write a script together for a short-lived TV series, which unfortunately is canceled before we can submit it for consideration.

David Grayson wasn't my only motivating force in high school.

Before I meet him, I discover rather unexpectedly that I have a crush on my friend Murray. I've known Murray peripherally since the third grade but we don't become intertwined with the same circle of friends until high school.

Murray chooses interesting activities, and his involvement draws my attention to these as well. It happens that one of Murray's favorite teachers is a black belt in karate and is instructing an after school karate course twice per week, so I follow him into the martial arts.

The style is Okinawan, called Goju Ryu, or "hard soft way." The tests for advancement, called Promotions, are twice a year and we go to Bellingham where the high ranking black belts from all the dojos (schools) in Washington gather to judge us. There are four belts: white, green, brown and black. In-between rankings are designated by stripes on the belt which are the color of the next belt up. For example, in my first promotion I earn two green stripes, taking me halfway to green belt.

My commitment to Goju Ryu far outlasts my crush on Murray, which ends rather abruptly. I call him on the phone one day, as I often do. Our conversation is normal enough, but this time I decide to speak up about my feelings. I muster up courage, my heart a thumping lump in my throat.

"Do you think, you know, that there could ever be anything more than friendship between us?" I ask.

Matter-of-factly, he answers "No. No, I don't think so."

I draw in my breath.

"Oh," Is all I can manage. "OK."

"Oh!" he replies in realization. "Oh, you didn't really mean…oh, I'm sorry. I had no idea you felt that way."

"It's OK," I reply. And oddly, almost instantly, it really is OK. I wish all emotions of that sort would dissipate so easily, like turning off a faucet. No harm is done to our friendship. With that out of the way, it may have even made us closer.

Murray may have motivated me to join karate, but he is not

what keeps me there. I earn a green belt with two brown stripes by the time I graduate high school. I am able to continue my studies through college and by the time I complete my bachelor's degree I have earned the first level of black belt.

Though the end of my school years also mark the end of my dedication to the martial arts, the balance, coordination, control of breathing, use of deflection rather than meeting force with force, and a general awareness of my body carry over to other aspects of my life, including horseback riding.

A less favorable activity first manifests in high school as well. I am sitting in science class one day, concentrating on the project at hand. I am thinking hard through a problem, and I'm insecure about whether or not I'm on the right track. As I pull myself out of deep concentration, I realize that I am absently plucking at the hairs of my left eyebrow with the fingernails of my left hand. I also realize, as I examine the short thick hair between my thumb and middle finger, that I've been doing this for awhile. Not just today, but in the recent past as well. Worse yet, I can't seem to stop myself from doing it, even when I become aware of it. Nor do I particularly want to stop. The activity satisfies some inexplicable psychological need.

I believe myself to be unique in this behavior, until roughly thirty years later I am informed that this obsession has a name: trichotillomania. It is a compulsive disorder defined as the irresistible urge to pull hair. I consider myself lucky that I am able to confine this subconscious fixation primarily to the eyebrows which I can paint on with an eyebrow pencil. The occasional eyelash falls victim, but mine are so thick the absence of a few is hardly noticed. Sometimes I attack other facial hair, most of which I can stand to do without anyway.

This revelation that not only is this behavior not singular to me but has a psychological identity is one of many that has helped me to realize that nothing we do, think or feel is completely unique. When I've considered looking into possible treatments, I've stopped myself, not because I don't desire to eliminate this behavior, but because I have concerns that it might be replaced by something even more destructive.

Chapter Fourteen
My Choice to Make

Biological transformations, hormones and psychological adjustments compile with increased scholastic expectations and social rejection to make high school a time of emotional turmoil. Boys who were once my friends have discovered that it isn't cool to talk to me anymore. I am attracted to several others who are nice to me and I consider friends but any romantic feelings are never reciprocated. The surgical procedures are failing to yield the results I'd hoped for, and the realization of the limits of medical science is starting to slowly sink in.

Up to this point, I have generally done as I'm told and tried to follow rules as best I can. I am the model patient and the model student, never deliberately causing trouble. I always try to do as my doctors ask, no matter how much it hurts, because that is what is expected of me.

But amidst all these other changes, I am beginning to question.

I am figuring out that authority figures are human, and that people whose words I trusted absolutely might be wrong. I am also discovering that life isn't always fair or just.

As I struggle to sort out and reconfigure the ragged bits that have been strewn out before me into something that makes sense, I am torn in different directions by what I've been taught to believe, by experience, and by others trying to open my mind to other possibilities.

My mother is Episcopalian, and for years I attend the weekly service with her. Sunday school isn't bad, filled with story telling and art projects. But any time I have to attend the service, I am terribly bored.

As soon as I am old enough to be offered the choice, I stop going. I can tell that my mother is disappointed, especially since both siblings have done the same.

My father is agnostic. His mother was devout Italian Catholic, but he and his brother did not adopt that faith and he only attends church on special occasions. So from an early age I am shown that religion is an option.

My greatest influence is the friends I have made upon entering high school. We are all social outcasts who don't fit into the typical high school categories such as jock, brainiac or even nerd. A few are coming to terms with their homosexuality, some are poor, and some have opted for a Goth appearance. Whatever the reason, we gravitate toward each other. A few of us have been acquainted since early grade school but are only now finding commonality and friendship. I am the academic over-achiever of the bunch, but that doesn't mean I'm the smartest.

Murray, for all his insecurities, becomes our leader and draws us into his line of study. His is a mystic and spiritual view of the world, for which the deity is a duality and whose guiding force is feminine. It is an earth religion, driven by nature and natural forces, in which the deities have a hundred names. It is known as Witchcraft, or the Craft, or by its modern term, Wicca. Murray and a few others form a coven which they call Treemist. For years, Murray has been intrigued by European folk magic, which he has studied with zeal, but has only recently formalized his beliefs and adopted Wicca. Nonetheless, he is well-read on the topic and excels at presenting his views in a way that make sense. He offers no absolutes and no threats of punishment for non-belief. I am eager to explore this other realm.

Wicca is an earth religion, basing much of its belief system on natural cycles and phenomena. The Pagan holidays correspond to the changes in seasons, sun and moon cycles and to events such as the celebration of harvest or the fertility rites of spring. It is a religion that emphasizes balance. There is no attempt by the forces of Good to rid the world of Evil. Rather, it is accepted that one cannot exist without the other. It is matriarchal, with the Goddess as the central figure. Mother Earth.

Wicca is a very personal religion. There is no doctrine and no equivalent to a Koran or Bible. I express Wicca as I perceive and experience it, but each participant experiences and defines it differently. It has elements of occult, but is not a cult. It celebrates the horned god, but he is not Satan. Wiccans do not believe in Hell.

Even though this is how my closest friends believe, they apply no pressure. There is no threat of being cast out if I do not conform. Instead, this group is defined by non-conformity. However, being a member of the coven will give me a sense of belonging and allow a more intimate bond with my friends.

I attempt to be up front with my mother about my intentions. I bring it up while riding in the car with her.

"I'm exploring the possibility of becoming a Witch," I begin tentatively.

She almost drives into a tree.

"I do *not* want you to become a *witch!* Promise me that you won't."

This isn't going smoothly at all.

I mumble some sort of acquiescence. I'm not sure what sort of answer I was expecting. As if she would say "sure, go ahead, dear. Explore whatever you like." Uh-huh. Episcopalians are pretty liberal as Christians go, but seeking approval to radically change belief systems, especially to one that is so misunderstood, is obviously too much to ask.

I decide never to bring it up again. I have been to church enough to know the lines. I can give the right answers to make people believe I am still Christian if I want to.

However, it is my choice to make. Christianity has no particular hold over me, except that to date it is all I have known. I embrace Wicca and join the newly formed Treemist coven.

Chapter Fifteen
Dancing 'Round the Fire

The coven offers friendship, warmth, acceptance, intimacy and commonality. We don't all get along all of the time. Even in such a small group there are politics and control issues as well as all the normal drama associated with being in high school, but we set all aside for ritual. We have to. If we cannot work together in harmony then our efforts are useless and our collective energy tainted.

I am just as happy gathering in one of our living rooms as I am gathering at the Circle for ritual. I crave the companionship and feeling of belonging. It is a safe environment for me, where I am not mocked, bullied or ignored. As the coven grows in number, there are times I wish our social gatherings could be limited to a smaller more intimate group rather than the whole crowd. I tend to fade into the background when a lot of people are present, but in smaller groups I am much more involved in the conversation. But as a general rule no one is left out, including me.

On ritual nights, we gather together however we can get there. Cars park in front of Murray's house, and flashlights guide us along the familiar path to our gathering place. Murray's family ignores our activities. Whether they agree or not, they are content to let us do our thing undisturbed. Murray has a fire going. The fire is ringed by stones forming a circle within the Circle. The heat of the flames is welcome on this chilly night and we gather in close. We are out of sight of the house and its electric lights are not visible to us, though we know it is a mere stone's throw away. We are surrounded by the darkened forms of tall trees, set well back from the flames and safe from stray embers. It is a dry clear night, hence the chill. It will be a frosty morning for sure.

We sit on blankets, and in the warmth of the fire we shed our winter coats. I pull out my pentagram necklace. It is a gift from Murray and I hardly ever take it off. Yet here in this haven is one of the rare times I expose it to air rather than carefully hiding it under my shirt.

The High Priest and the High Priestess are adorned in robes. Though we have exchanged greetings and pleasantries, we gather to begin a different purpose, joining hands and encircling the fire. There is plenty of time for socializing later. High Priest Murray takes an audible deep breath. On cue we join him, breathing deeply the crisp air and doing our best to avoid the wood smoke. Someone takes up a bodhran and begins to drum a steady beat.

Murray begins. "We gather here to create a sacred space."

The ritual commences and we create that space together. Invocations and purifications are the formalities, done at each ritual. Only when this is done can the real work begin.

I am nearly entranced, yet I am always aware. My voice joins the music and chanting. While some go deep into altered consciousness, I am never able to completely cross over. Maybe the fear of not being in control stops me. Or maybe that realm is not open to me.

It is now that we discuss our concerns and determine how best to disseminate the collective energy we produce. To what cause do we wish to contribute our constructive force? World peace is a waste. Our efforts a mere raindrop in an endless sea. An ailing relative, a favored politician, a just decision or judgment, protection for a traveler; any of these types of noble causes meet muster.

There is a plan by the city to sell a bunch of land to developers. While growth is inevitable, we decide to focus our efforts on tempering the amount and speed of the growth so that less destruction of natural places occurs all at once. We visualize a harmony between forests, wetland and population for the area in which we live.

Softly, deeply, our voices begin. Visualize…

The flames crackle as we dance. Around and around and around the fire. Our voices resonate, together, the chant intense, our mind focused on one purpose and our energy unselfishly directed. The drum beats, our feet move, our bodies twist, swayed by the spirit flowing through us. Louder our voices, faster our feet. Our eyes closed and unfocused, everything directed inward then outward. We pull it from the Earth, we draw it from the sky, we tap ourselves and each other. A log sparks, the drum beats, our feet strike the earth in rhythm. Our eyes sting with smoke. Our hands and bodies rise as our blended voices increase in volume pitch intensity until the pitch is almost a scream the drum is furious like thunder and then-

Silence.

It is intense, powerful, focused and draining. A deliberate redirection of energy by a cooperative collective.

We drop to the earth, grounding ourselves, bringing ourselves back to the reality of the chill air and the hot flames.

We take each others' hands again and formally end the ritual.

"The circle is open but unbroken. Merry meet, merry part, and merry meet again. Blessed be."

"Blessed be," answer our chorused voices. We break free of each others' hands.

A bottle of wine is opened. The unnatural crackle of plastic betrays one of our companions as she pops the lid off a store-bought fruit tray. I pull a loaf of bakery bread from its paper cocoon with a rustle and unceremoniously tear off the end. It is soft and fresh, separating easily if not cleanly. I pass it to the person on my right. Chalices and cups emerge to receive the wine. I pour myself half a cup. As if in tribute to my Episcopalian past, I dip the bread into the wine. It drips as I draw it out and bite into it. The wine-soaked bread melts in my mouth. Ambrosia.

Hours pass. Hungry teens devour edible offerings as the greedy flames feed on the corpses of fallen trees. We trickle out as our curfews or other demands require.

My clothing is permeated and I wear the smoky odor of the fire home with me. I don't mind.

Sometime after college I discover that the ceremony and ritual central to most religions hold little meaning to me, and I now consider myself "spiritual but not religious." However, being Wiccan helped me to recognize the connection of all things. The Force, Cosmic Consciousness, whatever name you put to it, I have seen it work and it is there for any who reach into it. Of course it does not manifest into the telepathic powers of Jedi Knights or the spells of Harry Potter. It is more subtle than that. But it can be used by those who know how to intercept and channel it. The Christians and Muslims do this through prayer. The Buddhists chant. This is Majick according to the Craft.

Even now, after all I've been through physically and emotionally, and as much as my belief system has morphed, I still believe in magic, though perhaps by a different name.

Chapter Sixteen
Rough-shod

Some horses are uncomfortable with being touched. When you reach out to stroke them, if they don't shy away completely, their skin tries to crawl out from under your hand. Over time, with patience and gentle handling, even the most sensitive horses overcome this. On the flip side, many horses are over-handled as youngsters and become pushy and spoiled. They have no respect for personal space and will shoulder into their handler or swing their butt around and knock into a person if something else catches their attention. This is usually not out of malice, but rather a failure on the part of the handler to assume a leadership role. The horse has not been taught that this behavior is inappropriate.

I do not come from a touch-feely family. Sure, I get hugs from my mother, but casual touching or hugging is not second nature to me. In fact, I have an aversion to being touched at all. Even a well-meaning hand on my arm or shoulder makes me tense up and want to move away. So I am like the horse that shies away from being touched.

Yet doctors and medical professionals touch me all the time. This is OK because they're supposed to. It is necessary for the work we are trying to do. They tell me exactly what they are going to do and it's professional and impersonal. I tolerate it like a horse tolerates a bridle and saddle; I've learned that this is the way it is and I might as well accept it. In this respect I am a model patient. I seldom fuss or fight, though apparently I bit a doctor once when I was very young. My mother told him that's what he got for sticking his finger in my mouth.

But for most everyone else, my sense of personal space is broad, like the proverbial invisible bubble around me. Outsiders and even friends are not to violate the bubble. I involuntarily repel casual touches like a magnet of similar polarity. The feel of a touch surprises me. If I have to endure the hug of a relative I barely know I am stiff and try to get it over with quickly.

I associate physical contact outside of the medical profession with friendship, intimacy and trust.

My friends are much more into casual contact and hugging, and are determined that I should learn to be more receptive to these as positive interactions rather than as threats to my personal space. They don't understand why I'm so resistant, and I don't understand it enough myself to explain it to them. Maybe it's because most of the touching I've endured has been professional poking and prodding.

My friends wear me down with compassion, perseverance and determination until I gradually come to the understanding that casual touches and friendly embraces, while they might reflect familiarity and affection, do not need to imply intimacy. Years later I am able to offer a hug if I think someone needs one, and will generally accept hugs offered to me with much reduced awkwardness. Even so, it is difficult to curtail some sort of reaction when touched unexpectedly, even when it is with the best intentions.

My friends successfully alter this behavior in a positive way, but there are other behaviors they don't try to change. My friends assume that I've had a rough time because of my appearance, and they don't want to add to the hurt. So they let me hurt them with my words and don't call me on it. I am not nor ever have been intentionally mean-spirited. Rather, I have a tendency to say what I am thinking, and often not in the most diplomatic way.

For example, since I have always been slender, growing up I have difficulty understanding how people can be overweight. One intimate friend definitely has a rounder figure than I do. I ask her about it, wondering if it is something she intends to do anything about. In my mind, I am being curious and helpful, completely missing or ignoring her non-verbal cues that such discussion is hurtful and therefore not welcome.

Like the spoiled horse shouldering into people, I run roughshod over my friends' feelings. This is allowed to continue until I eventually lose friendships without understanding why. I am left befuddled, unaware of the level of hurt I've bestowed upon them.

Chapter Seventeen
With Great Resolution

As my junior year in High School passes the halfway point, I've repressed enough of the unpleasantness of the previous surgery that I'm ready to try again. Or as my father insists, the doctors need to finance their yacht and desire the income from our insurance company. I am to have two procedures done this year, the first in early April with a follow-up in the middle of summer. This allows adequate recovery by fall, when I am to begin my senior year and will need to be able to focus on school matters.

Part one is to be the last of the structural reconstructive efforts, after which I am to be turned over to a cosmetic surgeon, who will attempt to manipulate the soft tissue elements of my face. I am looking forward to this, as I am optimistic that once he takes over I'll be on a more certain path toward symmetry.

The surgeons outline the procedures they feel are necessary, but ultimately the decisions regarding my surgeries are made by me and my parents. The doctors can do nothing without their consent, and I have always been a willing participant. The timing is usually dictated by what has come before. Sometimes the previous effort has needed time to succeed or fail prior to moving on or trying a different approach. The reconstructive surgeries are all considered necessary to regain some semblance of normal function, such as my ability to eat more effectively and breathe more normally. The insurance company doesn't contest because these procedures are considered to be a direct result of original teratoma surgery.

I never question these earlier procedures. They are just part of what I have to endure. My parents, as eager as I am to restore me to as much normalcy of appearance as possible, support me physically, emotionally and financially. I would imagine that it is the desire of every parent to have a child who is able to lead a normal life, and they always want the best for me. But I am never made to feel that they are ashamed of me. They are not and never have been.

As I begin the transition from the reconstructive phase into the cosmetic phase, the new face in my medical life is cosmetic surgeon Dr. S. His manner is subdued, thoughtful and quiet. He is kind, well-spoken and has enough of a sense of humor to put up with mine. He is proud of his medical jargon and uses it liberally.

He comes highly recommended by Dr. W, which my parents and I consider a tremendous endorsement. Despite my faith in his abilities, Dr. S has no easy task before him. My face lacks nerve, muscle, and a proper underlying skeletal structure, so he is being asked to create the illusion of symmetry without the foundation to build upon. He sees in me a professional challenge. I see in him a hope for normalcy at last. We are both optimistic, but he'll need to be quite the magician to pull off this illusion.

On April 4, 1983 I am admitted to the hospital, still primarily under the care of Dr. W. His associate, an amiable chap with a charming British accent, meets with me to write up the required medical history report and performs a pre-operative physical examination.

"Hello, Dawn," he greets me warmly. We know each other so are able to skip the formalities. "Are you ready for this?"

"Ready as I'll ever be," I reply. I genuinely like my doctors and am usually in a good mood while with them, even while nervous about upcoming procedures.

"Are you clear on what the procedure is going to involve?'

"Isn't Dr. S going to try a nerve transplant?"

"He's going to have a look at the state of the existing nerve to see what can be done," he clarifies. "A nerve graft is a possibility. So tell me how you're doing. How do you feel about this?"

"I'm kind of looking forward to it," I reply. "Well, to the outcome at least. Skip all the painful stuff."

He notes in the records that I have "mentally accepted my incapacity with great resolution over the years." That's doctor-speak for calling me courageous.

The plan for the initial part of the surgery is to once more cut, paste, twist, rotate, push and pull to realign the lower jaw as much as possible so that the teeth come close to meeting up when my mouth is closed. This time bone grafts for altering the structure will come from my hip. They will also try to reshape my chin to make it more symmetrical. Actually, I don't have much of a chin at all so in fact they will be creating one.

The hip graft placement goes as planned, and Dr. S takes over for his part of the procedure. He sets about exploring the seventh nerve in my left cheek, searching for residual function.

He does not meet with a great deal of success. It seems that he finds it chopped to little bits sticking out ineffectually here and there. However, the left side of my face is not completely devoid of nerve activity. He notices involuntary muscle spasms in my left eyelid and behind my ear.

I finish out my junior year with my jaws wired for a third time. Before the wires are cut and my jaws are freed once and for all, plans are already being solidified for the follow-up procedure in July. As I heal from this most recent bone grafting, I am gradually being handed over exclusively to Dr. S. The reconstructive surgeons have done all they can for the skeletal structure and realignment. This is bittersweet for me, as I like my doctors and feel an attachment toward them. It will be strange to not see them anymore, since they've been so much a part of my childhood. I actually feel sad about it.

But prior to part two of the procedure, I am to embark on a cross-country road trip with my dad.

Chapter Eighteen
The Long Haul

I sit on the broad black bench-seat in the cab of the Ryder rental truck, gazing out the window as the landscape rolls by as we head north on I-90 in Wyoming. A few feet away, my dad is behind the wheel, concentrating on the road. In a few hours we'll be in Montana. I have lots of time to think. There's only so much I can do to entertain myself as the truck roars along, since prolonged reading in a moving vehicle gives me motion sickness.

As I contemplate the trip so far, the AM radio is silent. We've grown weary of searching for a new station each time we drive out of the frequency range of the previous one, so the soundtrack for my thoughts is the rumble of the engine and the squeak and rattle of the cab as the tires find flaws in the road.

My maternal grandmother passed away in her home state of New Hampshire a couple of months ago. My mother's share of the inheritance included a modest set of belongings, mostly furniture, which my parents determined were worth finding a way to bring home.

My dad was making frequent trips to the Washington, D.C. area on job-related business, so at the end of his most recent excursion he flew to New Hampshire and rented the truck in which we are currently traveling. He loaded up my mother's entitlement which fills our ample truck to about half capacity. I'd flown over a week earlier from Seattle, visited relatives, and now I am accompanying him on the road trip home. I wouldn't mind sharing the driving, but I'm only just shy of my 17th birthday and the rental truck rules clearly state that "no one under the age of 18 is allowed to operate this vehicle." I suspect my dad may actually prefer it this way, and besides, it justifies frequent stops which benefit us both.

I had mixed feelings about taking this trip. I'd been in the midst of a phase in which I chosen to be at odds with my father, which seems to be fashionable for teenage daughters to do.

Growing up I adored my dad. I sat with him to watch football games and loved to perch on his knee during favorite television programs such as *Star Trek* and *The Avengers*. He was also my protector and I felt safe with him. Yet he has also been the disciplinarian. His quick temper and raised voice could be quite scary, though he has never been abusive. My rationale for being at odds with him may simply be that he is the closest thing I have to an authority figure to rebel against.

One of my friends grew up essentially as an only child since her sister is considerably older, and her parents seem more like friends to her. Her mom is the "cool mom" that seems more like one of us than a distant adult, and I have been envious of that relationship. My parents are great, but I've always considered them as parents rather than people I'd hang out with. Yet here I am, providing my dad with companionship on what would have been a boring and grueling drive alone. My presence helps to justifies the many stops at national monuments and tourist sites along the route. They make the trip longer, but much more interesting and enjoyable.

"Well, there, DC." My dad's voice cuts into my thoughts. It is not unusual for him to call me by the first two initials of the name on my birth certificate.

"Hmmm?" I reply, still distracted.

"Are you enjoying the trip so far?" he asks.

I snap myself back to the here and now.

"Sure." I turn to face him. He has his right hand on the wheel, the other arm laying on the arm rest of the driver's side door. I can't see his eyes through his sunglasses but I know he is watching the road. The sun has given us both healthy tans.

"Lots of interesting places to visit," I continue.

"The terrain around Devil's Tower is sure different from the movie," he comments.

"Yeah. No place for the mother ship to land."

The recent stop at Devil's Tower has been a highlight for me, as *Close Encounters of the Third Kind* is one of my favorite films. The realization that the terrain around this natural feature doesn't match what is depicted in the film is one of my early introductions to how Hollywood alters things for its own convenience.

The bag on the seat in between us catches my eye. It has a graphic depiction of Devil's Tower.

"Thanks for the T-shirt."

He nods but doesn't respond.

"We'll be home in a few days," he finally says.

"All I have to look forward to when I get home is another surgery," I lament. "Seems I barely got the wires cut from the last one."

Indeed, the swelling has only recently gone down and the scars are still red and itchy.

"The new surgeon comes highly recommended. Your mother and I are really hoping he does great things for you."

"I hope so too." Pause. "At least I shouldn't have to have my jaws wired again."

"I hope it's all worth it," he responds thoughtfully.

I look over at him and realize that I am studying the profile of someone I really don't know very well. Odd considering I've shared a house with him all my life. What's more, it's someone whom I know cares deeply about me, and who's company I find myself enjoying. We are getting along well, which is no small task considering we are spending thousands of miles cooped up together in a tiny truck cab. Even when the truck broke down on the climb to Mt. Rushmore, he didn't take his stress and frustration out on me.

At a busy truck stop in Montana I go into the restaurant for a sundae while my dad does some minor maintenance on the truck.

The waitress who serves me is stout, middle-aged and kindly but with a hardened edge. She sizes me up.

"What brings you here?" she asks me.

"Waiting for my ride," I reply, offering nothing more.

"You might have trouble getting a ride here," she cautions, but there is no threat to her voice.

I glance up at her, surprised. She thinks I'm looking to hitch! It strikes me as somehow fanciful. I am both embarrassed at her misinterpretation yet oddly smug. The adventurous part of me wonders what it would be like for a young teenage runaway to travel with truckers.

It occurs to me that she refers to my appearance when she says I might have trouble getting a ride here. Truckers are an odd lot. I am not convinced my face would make much difference to them if they were looking for merely a traveling companion. I am not brave enough to hitch a ride with a complete stranger, regardless. I am naïve but not stupid.

I am suddenly relieved that I really do have a ride waiting. I am glad that my destination and means of getting there are not in doubt, and I am glad that my traveling companion is someone I care about and trust. I deposit a handful of change on the counter as a tip. Considering the cost of the sundae, it is a generous percentage.

"I'm riding with my dad," I explain proudly and securely as I get up to leave.

She nods. "Have a good trip."

As I climb into the cab next to my father to resume our journey, it crosses my mind that my view of him may not be the only thing that is changing.

I wonder if he is realizing that his youngest child, third of three, is becoming a young adult.

Regardless of how interesting the journey has been, we are both eager to be home, despite the fact that my next surgical date is imminent.

Chapter Nineteen
Activity as Tolerated

It is late on a dark night in mid-July. My friends are laughing and joking under the amber light high atop a pole in Cora's large secluded yard. The huge house looms nearby, a diffused light in the living room indicating that her parents are still up watching television.

My mood is dark and brooding and I cannot share in the levity. In fact, I feel ignored. *Don't they get it? Don't they care?*

"You guys do realize I'm having surgery tomorrow," I finally interject, my long silence broken.

"Yeah," says Murray matter-of-factly. "What's the big deal? You do this all the time."

"It doesn't get any easier the more you do it," I retort. "It's horrible. I hate going through it."

"Then why do you do it?"

"Because there's still so much that needs to be done."

The others are silent. I cannot read their expressions in the awkward overhead lighting.

"So what do you want us to do about it?" Murray asks.

"Well, gee, maybe some support? I didn't think that would be too much to ask."

They probably all think I'm gunning to be the center of attention. Maybe I am, but maybe it's because I need to be.

It is the first time that I recall the necessity of these surgeries being called into question.

July 19th, 1983 finds me once again in an operating room. The primary purpose of this procedure is to graft a muscle from the inside of the upper left thigh into my left cheek. Ideally, this will serve two purposes. Cosmetically, it will help fill out the left side of my face so it won't slant downward quite as dramatically. Also, it is hoped that the muscle might take hold and allow for some partial reanimation.

Secondarily, there are some Steinman pins that need to be removed from my chin, which had been placed there two months ago during chin reconstruction. A Steinman pin is a very expensive stainless steel straight pin used as an orthopedic device.

Once again the old incisions are opened up and the skin of my face is peeled back. They shift things out of the way to make room for the muscle flap, as well as identify the source of the blood supply required to feed the graft once it is inserted. Having prepared the accommodations, the surgeons now go after the soon-to-be occupant.

I am told that there are three main muscles in the thigh and not all are needed. Time proves their assurances to be accurate, and even as a horseback rider I find I don't miss use of it. However, its absence leaves not only my most impressive scar to date but also a notable indentation on the inside of my upper leg. The scar is wide, running down my inner left thigh from the pubic area nearly halfway to my knee. It is visible when I wear a swim suit or short enough shorts, neither of which I wear often. However, my choice in clothing is not because I have any particular desire to hide it.

After the muscle flap is settled comfortably into place and appropriately fed, the two Steinman pins are removed from my chin.

The surgery lasts nearly 11 hours. That is one *extremely* long operation, and for the first time the insurance company doesn't want to pay for it. They don't cover cosmetic surgery, so my surgeons have to convince them that this is still directly related to my original condition and is considered reconstructive and not strictly cosmetic, despite the change in medical personnel. Thankfully, the insurers are able to be convinced.

For the first time in four surgeries, my jaws are not wired coming out of the OR. My post operative instructions dictate activity as tolerated and a soft food or liquid diet.

Activity as tolerated takes on special significance. I am active, and I can tolerate nearly anything, regardless of whether or not I *should*.

Still hobbling from the surgery but with most of the swelling abated, I take the goats I've been raising to the county fair with our school chapter of FFA (Future Farmers of America). I clean pens, climb rails, change water, groom my animals, take my turn sweeping the aisles, and all other duties associated with having animals at a public event.

My leg begins to hurt a little worse, but I try to ignore it and not let it slow me down.

By the time the fair is over, my thigh has started to swell up again. This doesn't seem right. The swelling should be going down, not increasing or even staying the same. I tend not to be an alarmist and prefer to wait it out, but my mother is beginning to panic. She takes me in to see Dr. S, who probes the wound. Finding nothing overly alarming, he takes the conservative course of prescribing antibiotics.

A week later the entire site has swelled significantly more, becoming hard and red and about the size a football. I am thinking that maybe my mother isn't over-reacting after all. This definitely isn't right, and my distraught mother hauls me, more willingly this time, to an after-hours emergency appointment with Dr. S. I have no fever, but this could be masked by the antibiotics. I experience no pain as he prods the wound, but since the entire area is numb anyway this doesn't tell him anything significant. The inflamed appearance is enough to convince him that admitting me to the hospital right away would be prudent, much to my dismay and my mother's relief.

The hospital staff immediately begin soaking the area. The next day, I am taken into surgery to open what has turned out to be a very large abscess and a marked amount of fluid is drained from the site. The procedure is over in a record-breaking 20 minutes. I awaken to discover that a drain, which consists of rubber tubing initiating in the cavity created by the emptied abscess, has been inserted into my leg. It is removed two days later. The fluid sample sent to the lab for culture is positive for staph so I am put on antibiotics for an extended period.

In order to try to prevent a repeat performance, *activity as tolerated* becomes a minimization of movement on foot, limited to 15 minutes at a time. I begin my senior year in high school in a wheelchair.

At first I see the wheelchair as a way to get attention, but I very quickly tire of explaining why I have it. After the initial barrage of inquiries, I am once again pretty much ignored.

However, having it does give me some insight into what it would be like to be confined to one. I discover just how many hills, steps, and ruts there are on my high school campus. In addition, my scrawny arms just aren't strong enough to get me around while I'm seated in the chair. On the rare occasions when someone gives me a push, we both agree that what I really need is a motor. But unlike people for whom a wheelchair is their only form of mobility, I am able to cheat. I can get out and push if I need to, and I find myself doing that more and more. The chair gradually becomes an elaborate way to carry my books. I celebrate when I am finally able to be rid of the thing once and for all, glad to hobble around on crutches instead. I recognize full well that some people don't have that option.

This time, I heal more successfully, and I soon return to my normal activities including animal husbandry and karate.

For the first time after healing from surgery, I am able to notice a significant change. The muscle flap has considerably filled in my left cheek. Even once the swelling goes down, I can still see that my face seems less bony and angular. It's a small step, but a significant one. All the pain and suffering is providing a pay-off, and I look ahead with renewed optimism.

Having to play catch-up from all the surgeries hasn't hurt me academically. I graduate high school with a 3.9 grade point average. I am not Valedictorian, however. In fact I am not even Salutatorian. No matter how hard I try or how high my ambition, there is always someone a little better or a little smarter than I am, which is something else I've had to accept with great resolution. This is not easy for me given that I am competitive by nature and strive to be the best at everything I do. Academics don't come easily; I have to work for my GPA.

I rank in the top 10 percent of all high school seniors taking the SAT test. Consequently, I am courted by colleges across the country. Therefore I am easily accepted into my selected university here in Washington.

Chapter Twenty
Alone in a Crowded Room

The first week of classes has arrived. I sit in the coffee shop off the main square at the university, killing time before my first class of the day. I am alone at my table, but the place bustles around me. It is morning, and people are loading up on caffeine.

Try as I might, I cannot figure out the appeal of coffee. I have to make it taste like candy for it to be even remotely palatable, but even then I get through half a cup and I'm done. Latte, my perfect solution, is not yet a household word.

I am not hungry. My dorm package includes a meal card entitling me to all I can eat three times per day. So I sit, taking in the crowd. I'm settling in to the new schedule, and the stress and anxiety of moving in, enrolling for classes, learning my schedule, and finding my classrooms is beginning to wear off as routine sets in. I can finally breathe and realize that I am excited to be here, beginning a new phase in my life.

I am still a stranger here. I have as yet made no friends. Occasionally I run into people I know from high school, but aside from recognition they are too busy making new friends and enjoying their new independent lifestyles to take much notice of me.

Around me I see people of varying ages, races, religions, and physical descriptions including those with visible disabilities, and it occurs to me that I am not some enigma here. This is a melting pot of diversity, as university campuses are historically known to be.

But what especially strikes me this particular morning is that though I've only recently turned 18, I finally feel like an adult, surrounded by other adults. I am not being treated any differently from anyone else in the bustling coffee shop. I am not sought out, but nor am I stared at or avoided. I simply exist here, like everyone else.

This is a day I'd been waiting for, though I never anticipated that it would just suddenly jump out at me and say "I'm here!" I feel a certain joy at being able to blend in, yet the dull ache of loneliness as well. I hope I can make some new friends soon. For now, however, I am alone in a crowded room. The uncertainty of the future in front of me is daunting, but the only way to go from here is forward.

I choose to attend this particular institute of higher learning for several reasons. It is removed from yet still close to home. Though my parents are generously paying for my education, I don't want them to go bankrupt doing so and this place is inexpensive as universities go. My brother graduated from here last spring. My sister is currently attending, but she will soon transfer to another university. My chosen career path is video and film production, but I can't seem to find a school which is both practical for me to attend and has a program suited to my goals. While not ideal, I can make the curriculum at this Liberal Arts college work. My dream has been to attend the American Film Institute in Los Angeles, but I haven't felt this to be a realistic option largely due to the expense.

Dorm life is an ideal transition for me, living away from home for the first time. I can walk anywhere I need to go, there are employment opportunities here, it's a reasonably safe environment, I don't have to prepare my meals, housework is minimal, and there is enough structure that I don't feel completely adrift.

For my first home away from home, I am assigned a room in an all-woman's dormitory. It certainly isn't my first choice but turns out to be my only choice. It looks very institutional, composed of metal and cement. Each room has enormous windows to the outside, but the views are hardly inspiring: another dorm, a sidewalk, a hillside.

I have one roommate and she is nice enough. I think they drew names out of a hat when making the match, however, as there are certainly no 37 levels of compatibility at work here. But I must say, we do get along all right, even though she is a fundamentalist right wing Christian activist handing out pamphlets and thumping bibles and I am still Wiccan. We don't talk about religion and politics much, but we do talk which helps alleviate the loneliness. Many times, we simply leave each other alone. We are both good students and neither of us are partiers, so on an academic level we are compatible and that's probably on what grounds this match was made. We like and respect each other, remaining roommates for the entire year, but once our sentence is served neither of us have any interest in keeping in touch aside from a cordial greeting in passing.

My coursework is pretty standard for an incoming freshman. Large crowded impersonal lecture halls are presided over by bored professors hashing over the same tired material. I struggle to stay awake in class, but unlike elementary school I cannot blame apnea; only late hours, early mornings and monotonous lectures.

My first job on campus is with the food services, but as soon as there is an opening I am hired by Media Services, which is responsible for making sure that professors have audio visual equipment in their rooms when they need to use it and operators when they need someone else to run it for them.

I am slow to make friends. Dorm life doesn't offer much socially for me. My roommate and I certainly don't hang out together outside our room and I have no way to relate to the groupings of people I see all around me who seem more interested in socializing than studying. But I would love to have at least a few people to hang out with. I visit my sister periodically but though she is helpful and supportive she has her own studies, her own friends and a boyfriend so not much time for me.

Gina, the Resident Assistant for my floor notable for her wavy red hair and flashing green eyes, is personable and makes an attempt to get to know everyone. As I pop in to ask her a question one afternoon, I see a photograph of what appears to be my brother's best friend sitting on her desk.

"Is that Gary?" I ask incredulously.

"Why, yes, it is," Gina replies. "He and I are dating."

Gina is a sophomore and Gary is in his fifth year.

"That's my brother's best friend!"

"Brian's your brother? Sure, I know him."

Thus begins one friendship. However, even though we hit it off fairly well, we are diverse in our studies and interests and though we chat periodically we don't spend time together outside the dorm. The age difference is only a year or two but still seems significant. She is a math major working toward her teaching degree, so I doubt I would fit into her circle of friends especially considering I avoid math as much as possible.

A couple of members of the coven have enrolled here, too, so this connection hasn't yet been broken. I visit them and we hang out sometimes, especially when Murray or another coven member comes to town to visit. I enjoy the time we spend together and am glad to be included in these social events, but as time goes by I feel more and more disconnected even from this group. We seem to be going our separate ways and pursuing different interests.

I am jealous of people who arrive at college with friendships intact, or who are quick to make new friends, and disappointed that the people I know from high school seem to have little interest in me or what I'm doing.

Meanwhile, I continue studying karate. The local dojo, or school, happens to be the hub in the region for my particular style, and also happens to be within easy walking distance from campus. I attend two nights a week plus most Saturday afternoons for the entire five years I remain in town.

Karate provides an outlet for frustration and a constructive outlet for my competitive nature. My goal of achieving my first level of black belt before I graduate gives me a focus and a path outside of academics.

It's a Thursday night and I have a test in one of my classes tomorrow. I thought about using it as an excuse not to attend karate, but frankly some physical exercise and a mental diversion are probably just what I need. Besides, with a promotion on the horizon I need to attend as many classes as I can. As I approach the old white church which has been converted into a dojo, I hear voices, thumps, yells and kiais emanating through the open door of the upper story. Some people get there early to do some extra practicing and warm-up.

I descend the outside steps to the lower storey, nodding a greeting to several of my fellow students as I enter. Two young boys, both already wearing gis, race past me. They are not even twelve and both have brown belts.

"Don't run!" The commanding voice of an adult black belt rings out, and the boys instantly slow to a walk.

I enter the building to the hum of voices and the creak and groan of the wooden floor above my head. I can see where posts and beams have been added for extra reinforcement. I recognize all the faces even if I don't know all their names. It's a good turnout tonight. I am inspired by the diversity of the membership: small children, college students, businessmen, housewives, police officers and even one man in his 70's who is moving right up the ranks with us.

I cross the basement floor to the small curtained women's dressing room and let myself in. I am welcomed by the occupants, each in various states of changing, and I greet them in return. I drop my gym bag on the bench, unzip it and pull out my neatly rolled gi tied closed by my belt, undo it, and proceed to undress.

"Where's Darcy?" I ask, taking mental inventory of who's there and who isn't.

"Family obligation," someone answers. "One of her kids has a music recital tonight."

I tie on my top and grab my belt.

"What about Jamie?"

"Here," says a voice as the person who owns it bursts through the curtain. "Got a little held up." She hurriedly begins to change, knowing there isn't much time left before class begins.

Darcy, Jamie and a handful of others are proceeding up the ranks at the same rate I am, which gives us a certain kinship. It is with this group that I feel the closest connection. The entire dojo is like a big family, and there is always a gathering in the kitchen after class for those who can stay to socialize.

My green belt securely tied and my hair pulled back into a pony tail, I and a few of the other women head for the stairs. I dread warm-ups most of all, but once suffering through those the rest of class will be interesting. I also securely know that I'll leave here tonight feeling much better than I did when I arrived.

Still, despite being a part of the dojo family, I don't bond with any particular individual and don't socialize with my karate friends outside of the dojo except on rare occasions. The men and women here have pre-existing relationships, families, and lives. I don't have enough in common with any of them outside of karate on which to build anything solid.

Surrounded by people everywhere, I find myself still hungering for more of a social life. I see a notice on a campus bulletin board for a meeting of the Science Fiction Fantasy Club (SFFC) and decide to attend.

Chapter Twenty One
Academic Pursuits

What can I say about the SFFC except that they make me feel welcome. Doesn't matter that I am strange, look different and am socially inept. So are they. We are all linked by our common interest in Fantasy and Science Fiction, hence the club's name. We are, for the most part, nerds, or at least share nerd-like interests and behavioral tendencies.

I am not into the technical aspects of hard science, fiction or not, but I like a good story. Many of my childhood writings are fantasy stories, with talking animals and unicorns. I was born the year the first *Star Trek* series originally aired, so by the time I was sitting on my dad's knee watching it with him, the show had already achieved cult status. I became a fan myself and a lifelong Trekkie. *Raiders of the Lost Ark* shares favored movie status along with *Close Encounters of the Third Kind.*

For the first time since being with the coven, I am invited to parties and social events. It feels good to be included even if going to parties is not a way of life for me. In fact, when it comes to alcohol consumption, I've been fairly conservative. I would drink wine with my coven friends, get buzzed and be happy. But I have never achieved the status of actually being drunk. At least not the kind of drunk you hear stories about or see in movies. Not stumbling-passing-out-puking-waking-up-with-a-hangover drunk.

The SFFC hosts an annual weekend event and all members are invited to the kick-off party Friday evening. I am glad to be invited and glad for the social opportunity.

Not sure where else to begin, I approach the bar to get something to drink. It's no secret that there is alcohol available, and one of our members is serving. However, I am underage and this is taking place on campus, so by law I am not allowed to consume alcohol and they are not allowed to serve me. Being one who generally has no problem following the rules, I am fine with this and ask for juice. I am served a tall cup of what looks like fruit juice, smells like fruit juice and tastes like fruit juice. It's quite good, actually, and I have a second glass. Then a third. Wow, this stuff is good! I feel tired, but it's been a long week of classes after all, with late nights doing homework and studying. I am sitting with some of the other members and it isn't until I stand up and try to walk that I realize walking has become inexplicably difficult. Yet I am so clueless that I haven't realized what is happening.

Since sitting is now easier than standing, I settle on the couch between Mick and Tammy, both juniors and both majoring in education. This placement is not accidental, since Tammy and I have become friends so I feel comfortable with her, and I happen to find Mick attractive. Mick has handsome features, long curly black hair and looks like he might have walked out of a Renaissance Fair. I have not expressed my interest nor do I intend to, but I certainly don't mind sitting next to him.

However, I am totally surprised and a bit embarrassed when I wake up and find that my head has been resting on his shoulder. I don't make an issue of it and neither does he.

They offer to walk me back to my room.

"Sure, thanks," I say, glad for the company, and the three of us leave together.

In the elevator, Mick says to me "I don't mind that you passed out on my shoulder."

I feel my face flush.

Tammy is smiling.

"I didn't know what I was doing," I said, though I am encouraged that he said he didn't *mind*. Does that mean that he might possibly be interested in me?

Then my thoughts drift elsewhere. *Passed out? Is that what happened? That implies that I am drunk! But how can that be? I haven't had any alcohol!*

Yep, I am still that clueless. Tammy and Mick are quite amused that they have to point out to me that the bartender might have heavily spiked my drink. I am literally stumbling home *drunk*.

Mick and Tammy aren't much better off than I. Even in my state I notice that they seem very friendly toward one another.

Later that week I meet up with Tammy.

"So are you and Mick together?" I ask.

"We're friends," she replies.

"That's it?"

"That's it."

"So if I were to have an interest in him I could pursue that?"

"I don't mind," she responds.

"You're sure about that? I don't want to get in the way of anything."

"Go for it," she encourages.

Not long later I catch up to Mick walking through one of the plazas and I decide to just go for it.

"Would you like to do something together sometime?" I ask hesitantly.

"Are you asking me out?"

I get suddenly quiet.

"Because if you are, the answer is no." His tone is firm but kind, if that is possible. "I'm flattered that you asked, but I'm not interested in you in that way."

"Ah, well, OK, then that's that I guess." I try to keep my tone even. Inside I am crushed, the sting of rejection seeping through me. *What did I do wrong? Am I really that unattractive and unlikable?*

Here I am, in college, never dated, never had a boyfriend, and only once or twice had a boy express any sort of interest in me. One of those times it was a mentally disabled stalker at the county fair. I was at first flattered by the boy's interest, but the genuine concern by the adults soon had me scared.

Within days of Mick's rebuff, I discover that he and Tammy are dating. I am not angry or jealous, yet nor am I surprised. I had seen it coming after all. Well, maybe I'm a little jealous, but it doesn't affect my friendship with Tammy and I am happy for them. Still, I wonder if she expressed no objection to me asking him out because she knew there would be no contest. Surely she knew that Mick was interested in her instead, and that it was unlikely he would be attracted to me.

I don't see much of Mick after that except at SFFC parties and events.

Another significant and long lasting friendship which forms via the SFFC is Sarah, a blond curly-haired Australian Whovian, which is another term for a *Doctor Who* fanatic. She, Tammy and a few of the others are close friends. Sarah is much more gregarious than I and is friends with pretty much everyone. She is studying theatrical costume design.

Sarah is there when I arrive and remains at the university until well after I leave. One might consider her a professional student. As long as she has her student visa, she is allowed to stay in the country, which requires a certain number of university credits. So I have one constant friend for nearly my entire college career. Though I wouldn't consider us close, we have a stable, reliable friendship.

After the initial selection of general university requirements, I have a difficult time choosing my major. There is no specific offering for film production or script writing. One option would be to find a different school, but I decide instead to force the choices of this university to fit my goals as much as possible. This does take a bit of innovation. I choose to major in Visual Communications with an emphasis on video production to provide me with technical skills. This offers a Bachelor of Science degree through the Technology Department. For the performance aspects, I take on Theater with an emphasis on directing as my minor.

I learn many interesting if now archaic skills while pursuing my Visual Communications degree, including burning plates for use on a printing press, black and white photography using actual film, and a programming course in Basic. I have trouble getting enthusiastic about the coursework because my sense is that except for photography I will not be using these skills again. This assessment turns out to be correct, despite having no concept of how soon the computer will revolutionize the graphic arts industry.

A television production course puts me behind a studio camera and at an electronic switcher. I enjoy the camera work but switching is too high-pressure.

When I need to use a computer, I have to go to the computer lab. Almost no one has a personal computer, there is virtually no Internet and email is all but non-existent. I cut my teeth on the Apple II series computers which notoriously crash. Thankfully I took a typing course in high school on actual typewriters, which proves to be one of the most practical classes I've ever taken.

While the Technology Department offers a certain set of skills, it is in the Department of Theater/Dance that I find not only like-minded people but also a set of life-changing opportunities. For it is amongst the would-be actors and actresses struggling for uniqueness and expression of their art and the nerdy-but-knowledgeable techies (those involved in the technical workings of a theatrical production) that I feel most at ease.

Chapter Twenty Two
Backstage in Black

I find myself spending more and more time in the Theater Department, taking classes with many of the same people. The Theater staff is small so it isn't long before I make my acquaintance with all of them whether I've had a class with them or not. I become friends with one of the professors, Adrian Pierce, and he allows me to use his office as a refuge between classes. When Adrian is there the office is generally loud and full of interruptions, so not fit for study, but it makes for entertaining and educational listening amidst the plumes of cigar smoke that frequently surround him. At first, I feel out of place in Adrian's odd entourage of undergrads, intellectuals, graduate students and faculty.

One afternoon I am sitting in the office opposite Adrian, trying not to inhale the second hand pipe smoke too deeply. Adrian's assistant, a graduate student who helps grade student essays, is with us and the conversation is lively. In an effort to fit in, I convey a situation that had amused me earlier that week.

"I could hardly keep a straight face!" I finish, hoping I've adequately conveyed the humor.

They look at me, exchange a look, and burst out laughing.

"Can you ever keep a straight face?"

I pause, my first reaction being surprise and hurt, as I generally do not find such comments humorous. I do my best to hide the hurt and to shrug it off quickly, offering a smile instead. It is intended only to be a bit of fun at my expense. I should be glad they feel comfortable addressing my appearance openly rather than having it be the elephant in the room. I realize that in order to fit into their world I must be able to accept this sort of ribbing. In other words, I have to at least try not to take myself too seriously.

I begin to attach myself to various theatrical productions in any capacity required, so it's a good thing that my punk/Goth friends helped me develop an affinity for black clothing. Having some in my wardrobe turns out to come in handy since stage managers, property managers, set movers, spotlight operators, light board operators, fly operators and all other stage hands and technical staff wear black during the run of a play or musical. The idea is that we become invisible in the darkness, outside the reach of the stage lights, offering the illusion that this all happens without us. Lights tinted by colorful gels wash the stage. Painted sets, furnishings and moving actors adorned with bright costumes and heavy make-up; these are the elements that are meant to be seen. If we have to be on stage in between scenes to move set pieces where there is no curtain to conceal us, we are meant to be ignored. We find our way in minimal light wheeling set pieces around, their final positions marked by glow-in-the-dark tape which has been charged by the stage lights during the previous scene. Then we fade away into the wings.

I do a lot of set moving. In one show, I help an actress do a quick costume change. In another, I give actresses a leg up onto a tall set piece and then have to spend the entire scene hiding behind it since there isn't time for me to leave the stage without being seen. I learn about fly systems, including spiking and locking ropes, and about hanging and hoisting the heavy black curtains called "legs" which block sight lines that would otherwise allow the audience to see backstage.

Light design interests me, so I enroll in the introductory theatrical lighting design class. The instructor is a graduate student who definitely knows his stuff, but it becomes very obvious that he has no clue how to teach it, at least not to someone like me who has no previous exposure. He hands out a light plot for us to study, and it might as well be written in code. Two weeks later I still have no clue what is going on, so I drop the course in a panic. I would eventually learn light design the practical way, by actually doing it, but not until after I graduate and start volunteering at a community theater.

Meanwhile, in a realm where most everyone wants to be an actor or actress, having a perennial techie is a luxury and I can find work in any show. The technical staff is generally made up of uncast actors or those needing experience doing tech support to fulfill class requirements. Usually, however, there is no class credit associated with the work. I enslave myself to the production for the experience, the camaraderie and the sense of accomplishment, and hopefully for the fun of it as well. Working in a theatrical production means late nights and sometimes finding time for class work becomes a challenge, but I am a night person anyway. Besides, I have an important role to play. I am wanted, appreciated and I belong. And I can hide in the dark.

I never fancied myself as an actress for obvious reasons. Not just because of my appearance, but because of my voice as well. It takes considerable effort to enunciate and to project. However, I find that I do enjoy acting when such opportunities are available, such as for class projects or in other situations in which my appearance doesn't matter.

Since I enjoy the opportunity to act, I am frustrated when one of the worst grades in my college career comes from acting class. I do my best to keep up my grade point average, but in this class I earn a very disappointing "C" for my effort. Our primary grade is based on a monologue that we have to perform. We have one rehearsal in front of the teaching assistant, who then gives us advice on how to improve. The assistant tells me that my rehearsal was spectacular, with just the right amount of emotion and inflection. However when it comes time to present the scene for my grade, I am told that my performance is flat. So if I interpret this correctly, my dismal grade isn't awarded me because I'm a terrible actress. Rather, it is because I peaked too soon. How often have we seen an actor "phoning in" their role? This means that he knows the lines so well that he just rattles them off without any feeling or believability. I see Tim Curry do this in a play in London, proving that it happens to seasoned and talented actors. For him, it could have been an off night or maybe he was bored with the production. For me, as a perfectionist and overachiever, I am devastated by the low mark. I discuss my frustration with the class instructor.

He is recently back to teaching part time after a debilitating stroke left him half paralyzed. His recovery has been remarkable, and he is walking and talking albeit with effort. When I look at his face I better understand what people see when they look at me. An eye patch covers his left eye and the left half of his face visibly droops. He supports his left leg with a cane as he stands before me.

"Dawn," he says slowly, struggling to keep his words clear through an unmistakable slur. He meets my gaze squarely. "You have a very good sense of comic timing. That is a gift. It's not something you learn. It comes naturally."

It's one of the nicest and most appreciated compliments anyone has ever paid me. I am thrilled and flattered, and I humbly thank him. Yet still my inside voice screams *so why did I get a C in your class???* Probably because I wasn't being graded on my stand-up routine.

As much as I know I can never make a career of acting, there is one play that calls out to the dramatist in me. It is titled *Tell Me That You Love Me, Junie Moon*, and portrays a troubled young woman whose face is disfigured by acid thrown by a psychotic boyfriend. It is a story about the humanity of outcasts.

In the latter part of the Director course at the university, each of us is required to direct a scene from a play. We hold a cattle call audition, dividing up the auditioners and also casting each other since most of us are aspiring actors and actresses anyway. One of the scenes is from *Junie Moon*, but I had no idea at the time of the audition what the play was about.

"Dawn, I've cast you in my play!" another director announces to me proudly.

Something in her tone makes me feel patronized, almost as if all the directors knew that someone had to cast me and she had gotten the short straw. It feels like being picked last for the sports team.

"Yeah, great, thanks," I reply, trying to sound enthusiastic. "What's the part?"

I have one line as a male bartender. Don't get me wrong. I am glad that I got a part. Even a little one. I dress like a guy, paint on a fake beard, and keep my voice as low as possible for my delivery. I swagger onto the stage deliberately not swaying my hips in an effort to seem masculine, and exercise that comic timing I seem to have a gift for. My one line is rewarded with a laugh.

All of the directors watch each other's scenes, and when I see the one from *Junie Moon*, I am puzzled. After the performances are over, I confront the director.

"Why didn't you consider me for the part of Junie Moon?" I challenge.

He looks befuddled, like a deer in the headlights. "Sorry. I didn't think…I didn't want to exploit you," he replies.

"That would have been my problem, don't you think?" I don't mask my disappointment. "That part is tailor made for me."

He'd cast his girlfriend instead.

So instead of a chance at a leading role I would have been perfect for, I'd had to settle for a pity-casting in a walk-on role as a male bartender.

Years later I see a community theater's production of *Tell Me That you Love Me Junie Moon* in its entirety. I find myself wishing I had known about the audition. The portrayal by the actress who plays the part lacks the passion of experience and the realism I could have offered.

Chapter Twenty Three
Restoration

My model horse collection, which grew tremendously in my middle school and high school years, has not been forgotten just because I've moved away to college. In fact, it takes on a whole new dimension. In the spring of 1986, I attend my first "live" model horse show in Vancouver, British Columbia, Canada. "Live" shows are so designated because they represent a gathering of collectors in a physical location, as opposed to, for example, sending photos of models through the mail. I send in my entry form, pack some of my favorite older and rarer Breyer models, and show up, having no idea what to expect.

Allegedly, the models are judged against one another as if they are real horses, on breed, color and gender characteristics. For example, if one of your models depicts an Arabian stallion in the color known as bay, he might be shown in three classes: Arabians, in which he is judged on breed type; stallions, where he is judged on masculinity, "presence," and whether if you owned a plastic Arabian mare you might find him a desirable mate for her; and bay, where he is judged on the accuracy of his color based on real life standards, as well as how well he stands out against others of the same color type.

As it turns out, I have some of the most valuable and collectible pieces at the show. However, they don't place well in their classes, and I am confused and deeply disappointed. The judge is Marney Walerius, who has since become legendary in collector circles. I find out much later that she has been Breyer's historian, and is largely responsible for researching and documenting the release dates and runs of many of the older Breyer molds and colors; information that was previously unrecorded.

"Your models are lovely, and I certainly would be proud to own them," Marney explains. "But in live show competition, condition is important. They have to look perfect."

"But how can anyone find models in perfect condition?" I counter. "They don't even come out of the box that way, let alone ones that have been in someone's collection for 20 years."

"Touch them up," she suggested. "A little magic marker on the ear tips, a dab of paint on a hoof rub."

"But won't that affect the value of the model? And how can they still be considered original finish?"

"It's a matter of degree. A few touch-ups here and there is one thing. Painting half the model is quite another."

Even with marred models, I still place very well in the collector's class, where age and collectability count more. But the seed has been planted to learn the craft of model horse restoration, and eventually my services are in high demand. At my 20th high school class reunion, I receive a special award for "still playing with the same toys." Apparently the organizers had found my model horse restoration web site.

The model horse collecting and showing community consists primarily of women and girls. Usually the only men are fathers and spouses, though some men and younger boys take an interest. The women are generally married, employed, and many have living horses as well. For some of us, however, the models are our substitute for our inability to own the real things at this stage in our lives.

For the better part of two decades I participate in model horse shows, taking on the roles of competitor, organizer and judge. I make a number of friends here, many of us questioning our sanity to one degree or another. I seem to fit in better amongst quirky people with hobbies outside the mainstream.

Eventually my interest and priorities shift from acetate and ceramic models to flesh and blood horses. I pay for my first Icelandic horse by selling off part of my collection and from money I earn doing model restoration, but that doesn't happen until 1997.

Nowadays I acquire living, breathing, hay-consuming Icelandic horses at about the same rate I acquire the model horses - between one and five per year. But all the models need is a space in which to stand and collect dust. The live ones are much more costly and much higher maintenance, making turnover more critical. And rather than collect dust, they roll in it.

In the meantime, my doctors have not forgotten me. Or should I say, I haven't forgotten them.

During the summer following my freshman year I partake in yet another episode of cosmetic surgery in my ongoing quest for facial symmetry. The exact date is July 20, 1985. I will turn 19 in a month.

My previous surgery involved the insertion of a muscle graft in an effort to achieve some animation on the left side of my face. The animation hasn't actually occurred, which is disappointing, but the graft at least succeeded in helping to fill out the left cheek area. Dr. S describes the upcoming surgery as a "balancing procedure." He will lengthen the nerve on the right side, fix my nose, insert a chin implant and add a bone graft to my right cheek. What is noteworthy about all this is the amount of work being done on the *right* side of my face. It is the *left* side of my face that is essentially numb and paralyzed. The right side, however, has fully functional muscles and nerves and has, to some degree, over-compensated for the absence of counterparts on the left side. So the muscles and nerve pull up on the right, even further emphasizing the asymmetry. Since he can't activate the left side, he hopes to craft the illusion of symmetry by decreasing the pull on the right side.

During the surgery, the muscle on the right side is lengthened and the primary nerve is loosened up so that it too will stretch. A freeze-dried bone from an outside source, probably bovine, is reconstituted and used to increase the prominence of my right cheek bone so that it will better match the left one. The graft starts out with the consistency of a wet noodle, making it easy to shape and contour, but later hardens to its natural solid state.

The chin implant is too big, so he pares it down. He inserts it through an incision made inside my mouth. The implant succeeds in filling in some hollow areas and gives padding to the previous bone grafts that provided a chin where I'd had none before. It is kind of rubbery, has some give and moves around a little. I can feel the rigid and rough line of the reconstructed jaw under and around it, but at least now there is some contour and fleshiness.

I get a nose job this time around too. Strictly for practical reasons, of course. I suppose I may have slipped in a small request to the surgeon along the lines of:

"As long as you are working on my nose, why not take down that huge Italian hump while you are at it?"

Nothing against my Italian heritage, but a little re-sculpting is in order. After all, Dr. S needs to try to widen the air passage on the left side to help me breathe more easily through my nose. And with my nose listing to the right he needs to make adjustments to make it appear straighter. Taking a little off the top helps him shape everything else better.

That's my story and I'm sticking to it.

The part of the procedure designed to increase airflow through my nose does not prove to be as successful. My left nostril is plugged most of the time and I cannot breathe through it, forcing me to breathe through my mouth. I can pull the soft tissue of my face over on the left side and unblock the passageway, which tells me that if I had muscle holding that up my airway would be clear. This is a minor inconvenience and I had no particular attachment to the success of that part of the surgery anyway. I am, however, delighted with my reshaped nose once the swelling subsides.

Overall I would rate this surgery a success. I have a nose I am happy with and I now have a chin. I can really see some positive changes and though we are nowhere near perfection I feel like we are headed in the right direction.

Chapter Twenty Four
Images

During spring term 1986, the Theater Department begins to buzz. Each fall term, the College of Fine and Performing Arts offers a "study abroad" curriculum, rotating emphasis between the different departments: Dance, Theater, Music and Fine Arts. The upcoming fall term has spun back around to Theater. The fly paper for theater majors, actors and techies alike, is that highly popular scene shop master and set designer Drake Glover is chosen as faculty advisor for the trip.

The agenda consists of spending two weeks in Italy, traveling by tour bus between Rome, Florence, Venice and Milan, then bussing to England where each person will have a home-stay in London for six weeks. The grand finale is attending the season of the Shakespeare festival in Stratford-On-Avon.

I am more attracted to the extensive home-stay in London than I am to visiting Italy. I've always been a bit of an Anglophile, probably stemming from watching imported television shows and movies, and who doesn't love a British accent? Students are expected to visit museums, art galleries, attend performances and have class discussions and critiques. This curriculum fascinates me, and I love the idea of getting college credit for exploring the sites and culture of foreign countries.

Another motivator is that I learn that my Australian friend Sarah, as well as several people I particularly like from the Theater Department, are signing up. Going with people I know makes the experience seem more comfortable than traveling with strangers. I send my parents the information and plead with them to let me go. To my amazement, they agree.

We land in Rome after dark in late September. Except for one brief stint over the border into Mexico, this is my first excursion to a non-English speaking country. I gaze in wonderment at other travelers, my ears buzzing with crowd noise and the blur of languages I can't identify. I do not stand out here. There is so much diversity a face like mine hardly warrants a glance. My gaze sweeps disconcertedly over the guards lining the public passageways, each touting a machine gun which I have no doubt they are willing to use. This is the first time I've been this close to militia bearing loaded weapons, and I am unsure whether to feel safer or more endangered by their presence. We have truly entered a different world, one outside our sheltering homeland. The red hair atop faculty advisor Drake Glover's tall stature is a beacon and I stay close, not wanting to get separated. This small band of 27 are my security. These are the only people I know. All other connections are on the other side of the world.

At breakfast the next morning, I observe the forming of social groups. Despite knowing several people and considering Sarah a friend, I don't feel comfortable inserting myself into any of them. Perhaps I am waiting for an invitation; an indication that I am welcome and wanted. None come, so I keep to myself. Yet going it alone the first day in this foreign city is too daunting, so as was so common in my childhood I once again attach myself to the authority figures. I form a trio with faculty advisor Drake and his mother-in-law, who has come along for the Italian portion of the trip.

Though we have a pleasant time, this alliance doesn't last long. On the second day, I wander off alone. I enjoy being with Drake but begin to feel the familiar anxiety that I am a tag-along or a pest. No one else invites me to join them, so I begin to feel sorry for myself for being the social outcast, which in turn makes me brooding and moody.

No doubt the isolation is born of my own insecurities, but going it alone does have advantages. I am free to do as I choose and am not bound by anyone else's schedule. It is in this way that I see many of Rome's galleries and cathedrals.

A week has passed. Darkness is settling in and the fog is rapidly closing in around us as we catch the foot ferry to Venice. It looks to be an interesting city, mysterious in the mists and the night. I once again isolate myself on the ferry, feeling the fog's prickling moisture on my skin, smelling salt water and diesel fuel and hearing the murmur of voices in several languages and the putter of the boat's motor. The harbors are littered with gondolas and motorized taxis. I am intrigued by steps that disappear beneath the water, slick with algae. The canals look green and murky. They will probably look less attractive by day, but in the low light they have a certain mystique.

With none of the tourist sites open and not much to see in the hazy darkness, a small group of us visit a bar. There isn't enough room at the table for all of us so I sit out, figuring I'd be the least likely to be missed. I listen in the best I can on the conversations, but my thoughts are turbulent and I struggle to put them in some sort of order. Days of feeling lonely and unwanted have taken their toll. I need to change something because I am tired of feeling like an outcast.

After awhile, I steel up my nerve and call Drake aside. He's had a few drinks, I am exhausted, and we are more or less alone, so the conversation should flow freely. It's a chat we both know has been coming. I can only bottle things up for so long before needing an outlet.

"I'm not sure how I fit in, Drake," I start awkwardly.

"How do you mean?"

"Theater...I mean, I'm obviously not cut out to be an actress."

"You'll find your focus," he encourages. "And when you do, there'll be no stopping you. You have so much energy. It boggles my mind how much energy you have."

I am flattered and humbled.

"You're a survivor," he continues. "But...maybe you aren't as independent as we all think."

"I can handle myself," I shoot back. "But I'm not sure anyone here really likes me."

"Well, I like you," he responds kindly, then adds "your path will be a tough one, but you are strong enough to handle it. In fact I'm least worried about you than I am anyone else on this trip." I glance up at him quickly, genuinely surprised. He considers me a moment.

"Though I wonder about your head sometimes."

Join the club, I retort silently. But his confidence in me lifts my spirits.

It seems like a bunch of clichés, but sometimes clichés are just what is required. When you're 19, they haven't become clichés yet.

"Hey, anytime you need to talk, I'm willing to listen."

"Thanks."

He also assures me that I'm not being a pest when I tag along with him, which makes me feel better about that.

My mood improves and my outlook changes, at least temporarily. Others in the group seem to take more interest in me after this and are friendlier towards me, so I wonder how much has all in my head in the first place.

My last day in Venice I am wandering the back streets where there are no tourists and very few people. I am here because I want to see what is off the beaten track; to catch a glimpse of what most visitors never see, and usually don't care to see. During my stroll, I observe dozens of cats, much more comfortable in the near-deserted areas of the city than around throngs of tourists. In one alleyway, I pass a pair of young girls cradling tiny kittens. Laundry lines hang over the liquid streets between residential windows, sporting sheets and shirts blowing in the sea breeze. It reminds me that this is a place where people live and not just a tourist destination.

As I examine postcards at a small corner souvenir stand, a man approaches me.

"Excuse me, do you speak English?" he asks.

I am startled at being spoken to. Except for the beggars and the pick-pockets, I am usually ignored unless I am purchasing something or suspected of being interested in purchasing something.

"Yes," I reply, curious.

"Do you mind if I take your photograph?" he inquires.

I stiffen.

"Why?" I respond suspiciously, as if I need to ask. I already know the answer but I am curious as to how he will respond. I look him over more carefully now.

He is dark haired with a mustache and beard, maybe around 40. He carries an expensive looking camera with a long lens and wears a couple of camera bags that give me the impression this may be more than a hobby for him.

"I find your face very interesting," he replies, looking straight at me as he says it.

Well he doesn't mince words. I am not sure whether to feel flattered or insulted.

"Yeah," I grudgingly acquiesce. *What's the harm?* "OK. Go ahead."

Then I ask him "Where are you from?"

"Los Angeles," he replies.

"Cool," I say, envisioning myself as a Hollywood scriptwriter someday. "I'm from Washington. Near Seattle."

He nods acknowledgement, frames the shot, and I stand for him silently as he snaps it off.

With his task complete it becomes obvious he is not interested in conversation and he hastily moves on. I am slightly disappointed by this as I would have like to have learned more about his intentions. But I am to him merely the subject of a photograph. I might as well have been a gargoyle perched amidst the surrounding architecture for all the interest he took. Well, at least he asked my permission, and flattery mixed with curiosity had edged out any tendency toward insult.

We'd been warned before we left that Italian men have few boundaries when it comes to physical contact with women, even on crowded streets. I am not sure whether to be relieved or disappointed that my face helps to spare me such an encounter. While yes, I would definitely have felt violated, my romantic imagination suggests I might have been flattered to be regarded in a sexual way. So I find it ironic that the only time anyone in Italy outwardly takes any notice of my appearance, it's a fellow American wanting a photograph.

I regret not asking if he had a deeper purpose in mind. I imagine the photo of my face hanging in some private Los Angeles dark room, perhaps being used as a reference by a Hollywood make-up artist. *Probably for some horror film*, I muse dryly.

Chapter Twenty Five
Depictions

It is a lazy quiet Friday and we've just finished with class, which is held in the upstairs room above a pub in London. We've been in London for several weeks now, and I've gotten to know my way around on the tube system pretty well. My home-stay is a self-contained flat just above our elderly hosts, which I share with one other travel-mate in the suburb known as Harrow on the Hill.

The printed class agenda suggests Queen's Gallery, but I don't feel like tackling yet another gallery and giving myself a headache looking at art. I'm pretty much galleried out by this point, so I proceed directly to the Science Museum, where I can give myself a headache reading labels in the Medical History sections instead.

The Science Museum contains seven floors of exhibits and I've been tackling them a few at a time. Free admission makes frequent returns possible. I enter near the now-familiar main hall, where the banks of windows that climb multiple stories to the high ceiling bathe the room with natural light even in winter's gloom. It houses huge steam engines and smells of metal, machinery and preservation. The tapping of footsteps echoes on the hard floor, blending with the chatter of visitors, the hum of sound effects and the tinny recorded exhibit explanations to create a barrage of white noise. Today's educational selection is located on the top two floors, so I make straight for the silence of the elevators. As I step off at the upper-most floor, I am amused by the identifying sign that greets me: "The Wellcome

Museum of Medical Science History." While I realize this section is named for Henry Wellcome, I smile wryly as I consider that I hardly find anything to do with medical science very welcoming. The word "welcome" implies warmth and pleasantness. My connotations for the subject are more cold, dark and painful. Too bad the guy's name wasn't Frost. Or Killjoy.

It's not that I find the subject of medical science or medical history distasteful. Rather, I find it fascinating, if macabre at times. Since England has deeper ties with ancient civilizations than the United States ever could because it is a much older country that colonized every continent, I am optimistic that its artifacts and depictions will provide me a broader historical perspective than I can find in my home country.

It is quieter here on the upper storey, with ceiling tiles at a normal height and thin carpeting helping to absorb sound rather than rebound it. This exhibit is also much less populated, and the atmosphere is more like a library than a recreational area. While the subject matter may not be warm and cozy, the air temperature forces me to remove my winter coat and carry it around with me. I have yet to learn to take advantage of the coat check, or "cloak room" as they call it in England. Besides, it's all the way in the basement.

As I peruse the various exhibits depicting how medical issues were handled by more primitive cultures, I am intrigued by the section detailing the practice of feet binding on young women in China. I recognize it as a brutal and prolonged form of cosmetic surgery, in which an alteration is made to the natural human form in the name of beauty.

When a girl in China reached the age of seven, the foot was bound in such a way as to prevent it from growing anymore. It tried, but merely ended up broken and misshapen. Children made to suffer through this found it painful for about a year until nerve damage rendered the foot blissfully numb. Small feet on women were considered attractive and parents believed they had to subject their daughter to this torture in order for her to be able to marry well. From the parents' point of view, they did what they thought best for their child and for the prestige of the family, just as most modern day parents would do whatever they feel is necessary to give their child a good life.

Yet I look at foot binding with my modern day perspective as an unnecessary brutality. I've certainly been carved on by surgeons and endured much pain and suffering in the name of cosmetic improvement. Nature altered my form, but medical science has been trying to put it back the way it is supposed to be. My parents made the choice for me at first, but by the time I was old enough to have a say, I've been conditioned to believe that my face should be as symmetrical as possible. While I may not be able to achieve beauty, I strive to be less unattractive. Might a young woman in the future look at my sort of procedures as brutal and unnecessary?

Since foot-bound women could barely walk, the poorer classes were unable to partake in this practice as they needed their women to be able-bodied. I view these as the lucky ones, but for them it reflected their inferior working class status. Many women whose feet had not been bound wore elevated shoes to hide their "large," unattractive and embarrassing appendages under their gowns. I understand the desire to hide what one perceives to be one's less flattering features. I often half-seriously consider wearing a veil in public. Or a kerchief that covers my nose and mouth, like cowboy villains wear in the movies. With just my eyes exposed, the abnormality of my face would be hidden. The skin below my left eye is slightly droopy, but a passing glance wouldn't notice. I'd consider a burka, but my figure is nothing to be ashamed of. But instead of staring at me because of my distorted facial features, people would stare at me because my face is covered. Curiosity knows no bounds.

For a Chinese man, it was a sign of wealth to be able to afford to have a wife who was crippled and unable to work on her feet. At least I will never have to worry about being considered a trophy wife. Anyone who marries me will do so in spite of my face, not because of it, and I'm fine with that.

The *Glimpses of Medical History* gallery is one floor down, and contains dioramas as well as full scale reconstructions depicting various medical procedures at various points in history. I am made more uneasy taking in these re-creations than I was when viewing life-sized portrayals of torture in the London Dungeons which I'd visited a week or so ago. The Dungeon depictions, though monstrous and sometimes graphic, seemed somehow distant. I had nothing to relate to, and the piped-in sound effects and screams made the atmosphere seem all the more fake. Here, on this quiet well-lit fourth floor, my stomach knots, my breath shortens, my body stiffens, and I shift my feet uncomfortably as I cast my eyes over the full scale replica of a 1980's operating theater. There is no blood, no sounds, and none of the familiar smells to trigger memory, yet I see the same machinery, similar instruments, and the technicians and staff dressed in familiar scrubs. It doesn't matter that the scene is set for open heart surgery. In my head I hear the beeps of the monitoring equipment, the clank of instruments, the hum of voices, the rush of my breath and the drum of my heart. I study the mannequin lying on the operating table under the surgical drapes. I feel a shiver up my back as I recall the icy metal slab and the chill of the surrounding air. *That's what I looked like. That has been me.* For a moment I am gripped by memory and imagination, staring in morbid fascination. I shake myself free of my disturbing vision and move on, though the impact of it remains with me.

Chapter Twenty Six
Empathy

My visit to the Science Museum's exhibit isn't to be my only brush with modern day hospitals this trip. The following Sunday, I learn that Michelle, one of my fellow travelers, has been admitted to a working London hospital with a severe throat infection. Her condition is described to us as silent, sore and swollen. I react with instant concern and empathy and I press Drake for more information. He tells me how to find her and reveals that this is her first time in a hospital in known memory. *She must be so scared!* I conclude. Being in the hospital is bad enough, but in a foreign country away from the support of your family would be terrifying. *At least it's an English-speaking country.* For me, going to visit her is not an option. It is an obligation.

The outside air is cold and damp, spitting on my flat mate and I as we traverse the overflow car park to the Lister Isolation Center of Northwick Hospital. I am filled with a sense of duty and a hope that I can make someone else's day brighter.

"They're not kidding about the 'isolation' bit, are they?" I quip as we notice the solitude of the building, sitting at the far end of the overflow car park, well separated from the rest of the hospital complex. We both laugh. But as we approach the building, the inevitable sense of dread creeps in.

We push open the glass doors to a wave of heat which feels good at first as we transition from the winter dankness, but it quickly becomes stifling. I am assaulted by familiar hospital smells and sounds, the antiseptic air invoking a feeling of uneasiness. For me, hospitals have little association with anything positive, so even though there is no particular haunting memory that replays in my mind, I'm left with a sense of general unpleasantness. I take a deep breath, trying to dispel the tension. *I am free to walk in, free to walk out. I am not trapped here. This is not about me.*

Ignoring my own discomfort, we follow posted signs directing us toward the section for infectious diseases, which puts us nearly at her door. Michelle has been diagnosed with a strep infection which is deemed highly contagious so she is set up in a private room. Before we are allowed to enter, we must strap face masks over our nose and mouth and pull booties onto our shoes. We are also required to don plastic aprons which seem to have little practicality.

When we walk into her room she seems in good spirits. Drake is with her, which may help explain her jovial mood.

"Hi!" she greets us brightly if hoarsely as we enter. There is no doubt she is genuinely glad to see us. Drake casts an appreciative smile our way. A flash in his eyes says *I knew you would come.*

In Britain's socialized health care system, a private room is an unusual luxury, or at least one that comes at an extra cost. As I make a quick assessment of the room, luxury is not a word that comes to mind. The walls are drab and bleak, there are no windows, the furnishings are plain, and it's as if a giant vacuum has sucked out all the color. There is no television, not even the blipping displays of monitoring equipment since her condition doesn't warrant its presence. It's a small room, not claustrophobic yet no bigger than it needs to be. The bed, tilted so its occupant can sit up, tucks head first against the back wall and takes up the majority of the floor space. Yet somehow, magically, the tiny room manages to accommodate all of us including the occasional visiting nurse.

"How are you feeling?" my flat mate asks.

"Better than yesterday," Michelle responds.

"That's not hard from what I heard," I add. I notice the IV inserted into her arm and try not to visibly wince as a phantom needle pricks my arm with a twinge of sympathy pain. I stop myself from rubbing the equivalent area on my own appendage. *It's not you lying there this time*, I remind myself, trying to dismiss the discomfort without losing the empathy.

I know what it's like, to be lying there. I remind myself that this is why I am here. Because I can offer something that maybe no one else here can- an understanding of what she is going through.

And I understand the importance of visitors. Having visitors means more than just having company, though in such a bland environment I would guess any stimulation at all is welcome. Visitors mean that people care about you.

I ask how many people have come to see her already, and am disappointed to learn that she has had only four visitors that day, including us. I hope that others from the tour will realize how important this is and make at least one appearance.

We stay and chat for about two hours, well after Drake departs. I leave with a promise to provide Michelle with some of her favorite chocolate bars, even though she is still on a liquid diet. I feel bad that she will be alone, but happy that I was able to brighten her day, and it gives me a warm sense of worth.

I know and like Michele from our association in theater, so she is not a stranger to me, but I would have made this visitation regardless of who in our group had been hospitalized. However, what brings me back to see her repeatedly is that she makes me feel welcome. My outreach is rewarded with appreciation.

The next morning after an abbreviated class session, I pick up a get-well card and the promised chocolate and return, solo this time. She is alone and happy for the company. I present the chocolate.

"You brought it!" She brightens noticeably.

"Here's your incentive to get back onto solid food," I said, handing it to her. She smells it longingly.

I feel wanted, even needed, which has been rare so far this trip. We sit and play cards, chatting away as much as her voice will allow, until her boyfriend Sean and another friend show up. We all greet each other pleasantly, but I quickly realize that my presence is about to take a back seat. My purpose has been served, her need for me expired. She has other company now, people with whom she shares a deeper intimacy. The familiar sense of being the odd person out slinks back in and I feel more like an intruder.

"You don't have to leave," Michelle insists as I make ready to depart.

"It's ok. I've got stuff I need to do," I maintain. "But I'll be back. I promise."

At my next visit, the staff has temporarily removed Michelle's IV, giving her a freedom of mobility she hasn't had in days. She is restless and bored, which comes with starting to feel healthier. Someone has brought her some books to read, but there is little else for her to do. I don't know how she stands it- I'd literally be climbing the walls. We indulge in a game of cards to pass the time.

The ward as usual is overly warm, and I've had to strip out of my winter layers.

"I haven't seen outside in days," she reminds me.

I glance around her windowless vault.

"You're not missing much. Damp. Cold. Typical London winter. Not so different from home actually."

"My home-stay is so cold," Michelle laments. "I'm afraid I'll just get sick again." She is scheduled to be released in two days, once she is able to eat solid food and take oral antibiotics.

"I'm sure they'll keep you warm enough," I assure her, hoping I am right. I realize in this instant how lucky my flat mate and I are. Not only do we have our own space, but we've been encouraged not to be frugal about use of the utilities. Many of our companions have a room in a house or even a bed in a shared room with families who appreciate the small bit of income hosting a foreign student brings in. Families on a budget can't afford high heating costs.

When Drake arrives a few card games later, the conversation becomes three-way and is light-hearted and entertaining. Most importantly, I am comfortable and do not feel compelled to leave.

When I walk through the door for my next visit, I am dismayed to see Sean and another friend already occupying two of the chairs. I have enjoyed the one-on-one chats and card games involving just the two of us. I prefer to be the central focus rather than being on the outskirts of a small group. However, Sean finds me a chair and offers me a seat, welcoming me. I begin by mostly just listening. Sean is a witty guy, and this is a theatrical group after all, so the conversation is interesting and entertaining. Gradually I feel more comfortable joining in when I have something to add, weaving myself into the social blanket. We are here for a common purpose; the support of a comrade in need. A disappointingly small fraction of the 27 in the tour group have made an appearance or offered Michelle any sort of sympathy. I belong to the conscientious few who have. *I belong.*

On the evening of her release, I call her home stay to make sure she has made it home all right. A woman answers.

"Did Michelle make it home from the hospital?" I inquire awkwardly.

"She did. May I ask who's calling?"

"Sorry, this is Dawn, one of the students on her tour. Is she available to talk?"

"I'm afraid not, she's sleeping right now. Can I take a number and have her ring you back?"

"No, that's not necessary. I mostly just wanted to make sure she made it home all right."

"That's very kind of you."

Several nights later, on the way home from attending a theatrical performance I'd attended on my own, I meet Michelle, Sean, and one of their friends on the tube. I am heartened to see her up and around, looking a bit gaunt but overall happy and healthy. She lights up when she sees me.

"I would have called you back," insists Michelle, pretending to be angry. "How come you didn't leave a phone number?"

"I didn't need for you to call me back," I reply seriously. "I mostly wanted to make sure you got home OK."

It is heartening to be greeted so warmly and to be as well received as I am that night on that tube. Someone is actually glad to see me. Someone cares.

I continue to explore London on my own. While I am certainly on better terms with Michelle and her friends and am more comfortable around them, I don't assume any special status just because I've visited the hospital. Friendship doesn't always work that way. Besides, I'm so used to being on my own schedule that by now I actually prefer it that way

Chapter Twenty Seven
Solitude

On Saturday November 22, 1986, I am sitting in a youth hostel in the walled city of York. The Study Abroad program has ended, but as planned from the outset, I have stayed on for an additional period of exploration. I've activated the rail pass I bought well before leaving the United States and this is the first stop on my solo journey. This morning I was in London, stuffing things into my suitcase, only to spread them out again upon arriving here.

The thought that I am now totally on my own in a foreign country should seem daunting, but by this time I am so used to it that I hardly notice the absence of my tour companions. In fact, I feel liberated. I am completely free of any obligation save my flight from London in two weeks. No guilt, no feelings of rejection, no requirements to be a certain place at a certain time or visit a certain gallery or museum. The twinge of longing that tempted me to fly away home with the majority of the tour attendees is dissipating. I've embarked on a great adventure and I'm going to enjoy it.

I have chosen to spend this time exploring the north. After a day of visiting York's museums, I succumb to a whim and catch a train to Scarborough, a small town on the wave-savaged coast. The town itself has little to offer this time of year. Its carnival rides are mostly silent, and the game barkers huddle inside their booths with their blankets and space heaters. I make my way upwards, to the ruined stone castle and beyond.

I stand atop a cliff, gazing out at the North Sea and reveling in the solitude. It's a burly wind, tossing the water into monstrous waves and forcing me to widen my stance to stay upright. I am completely alone up here, for I am outside the tourist season and the locals are too sensible to be out in this weather. The gale blows icy cold, whipping hair into my eyes and making my nose run. I bear the brunt of it a few moments longer, the assault on my senses reminding me how alive I am and how far I've traveled to be here.

I may be feeling free and alive, but I am soon also feeling frozen, so I make my way back down to the near-deserted streets of this seaside carnival town, seeking out a place to warm up. Though the train doesn't leave for another hour or two, Scarborough is the end of the line, so it sits at the station waiting and warm. Passengers are allowed on early, so it is there I find refuge.

What would be Thanksgiving Day in America finds me on a southbound train to Glasgow, Scotland. I've just left Inverness, where I'd enjoyed a haggis picnic en route to Loch Ness. As I stare out at the moors we are rumbling through, I think about my family, imagining they'll miss me at their Thanksgiving dinner table. My mother will undoubtedly make specific mention of me as she says grace, praying for my safe return. This gives me comfort. As the train pulls into the Glasgow station I surprise myself by feeling grateful to be back in a large city again. Normally I prefer the peace, quiet and openness of rural settings.

The habit of visiting art galleries and museums is so engrained by this time that it just seems the natural thing to do as I explore each city. However, I have had enough of cathedrals.

December arrives in Edinburgh the same day I do. I spend a few days there, which is enough to make the acquaintance of other student travelers who are staying at the same hostel. We visit the pub as a group and watch videos together in the hotel's main room. Yet it seems that just as things get going socially, I say farewell and leave. The irony is not lost on me, but there are no attachments to be made here.

The realization that I am now headed home doesn't hit me until the train is rolling south. Though I love it here, I've been a long time away and am feeling homesick. The five hour train ride lands me back at Harrow and Wealdstone, where the pouring rain soaks me and my luggage on the short walk from the train station back to the flat where my former hostess has graciously allowed me to resume my stay. I wish I were flying out immediately, but I have to wait another day. At least the weather for my last day in London is sunny and clear.

As glad as I am to be home, especially being able to spend Christmas with my family, it doesn't take long for the novelty to wear off. The university is on winter break, but I need to scramble to find an apartment before the next term begins in January. After two years of living in the dorms it's time to try my hand at running my own household, and my parents are willing to provide financial help. Finding a house or apartment for fall is nearly impossible, but by the second term people have dropped out or moved so there are more vacancies. I settle into the upstairs of a duplex: one bedroom, kitchen, bath, living room. I have no roommate, I have loan of a car, and I am allowed a cat. My parents are moving to Virginia for a couple of years, so they send their portly orange yearling cat Fizzbin to come live with me. We spend the next 18 years together and we inhabit that duplex until the end of my college years.

Living alone is peaceful, but it can also be lonely. People don't have cell phones or personal computers to connect them, and I am a person who needs to be connected. I sometimes feel very isolated. It is possible to run up hundreds of dollars in phone bills just calling friends who live out of town, which is money I don't have. Postal mail is the only way to send someone a message but a response might take days or weeks.

I am within walking distance of the university, and the karate dojo is on my regular path, so it is easy for me to continue my martial arts studies. My dojo family, my SFFC friends, and the people I've met in the Theater Department continue to provide me with much-needed companionship and social interaction.

Chapter Twenty Eight
Epic Fail

I turn 21 in August of 1987. I am covered by my parents' insurance until age 22, so if more work is going to be done we will need to do it in the next year. Changing health plans will likely be problematic in terms of getting approval for future procedures.

Dr. S orders a nerve test and I dutifully show up for it. An electrode is inserted into the muscles that close the eyelid on the left side. I have never in my memory been able to blink the left eye independently and it does not close all the way. I do have independent control of my right eyelid, however, and thankfully the left eye has a slave reaction to that. In other words, I can close the right without closing the left, but I cannot close the left without closing the right. Indeed, the electrode records no electrical activity and no voluntary motor activity. Same result when inserted into the muscles below the eye.

The technician tries to stimulate the facial nerve at the angle of the jaw with the needle in two locations. No response. Basically, the muscles around the eye have wasted away due to damage to the peripheral nerve supply.

While it doesn't tell me anything I didn't already know, this test is preliminary to a much larger procedure to take place only a few weeks later. My surgeon needed to know what resources if any he has available to him.

While all previous procedures have been designed to improve function and enhance the illusion of symmetry, this particular surgery is for *me*. My surgeon and I have designed it specifically to address areas where I want to see improvement, so I am particularly excited about the intended outcome.

I have selected three areas where my surgeon feels he can successfully make a positive difference. The first is to transfer fat from my abdomen to the left side of my face to fill out the hollow area between my cheek and neck. The transplanted bone which simulates a jawbone protrudes in an abrupt angular fashion, and I want it to have more curvature to better match the right side. The fat will come from the omentum, which is the membrane protecting the abdominal cavity. I don't have a lot of fat to spare, but not much is required. I'm sure if it were an option we could find plenty of willing donors.

The second goal is to sew together part of my upper and lower left eyelid to decrease the size of the opening in hopes of making my left eye appear similar in size to the right eye.

Thirdly, another bone graft will be added to my right cheek to build up the cheek bone to match the constructed one on the left.

When the surgeons confront me with the idea of removing pieces such as muscle, bone or fatty tissue from one location and transplanting them to my face, I respond with passive acceptance. If this is what is necessary to accomplish the desired improvements, it is fine by me. The scars I bear in locations other than my face are largely hidden, and even when they are visible I am not self-conscious about them. So I allow my body to make sacrifices which could improve the one part of me I am self-conscious about.

I admit myself to the hospital late on a Friday, bouncing with nervous energy and apprehension. It feels odd to come to the hospital alone. In the past, my mother has accompanied me, but I'm legally an adult now, so this is the first surgery for which I've been able to sign my own paperwork. It's not like

I've never done anything like this before. I'm a hospital veteran and a world traveler. I can handle this. Besides, my mother will be here soon enough and will help with the aftercare.

I am spared a completely sleepless night by the exhaustion of jet lag, having just returned from visiting my parents who are temporarily living in Virginia, only to awaken in the darkness tense, nervous, and without a clock.

An hour before the gurney, the needle arrives to take blood for tests. I have miraculously rediscovered a sound sleep when the vampire arrives to put an end once and for all to my peaceful slumber. They have no trouble withdrawing what they need.

I chat pleasantly with the operating room attendant sent to fetch me, partly because I have an amiable nature, and partly because such discourse keeps the apprehension at bay. I am abandoned in pre-op, surrounded by its smells of antiseptic, anesthesia, and whatever else creates the indelible odor unique to hospitals. Left alone to wait, I have only my thoughts, memories and anxiety. I dread what comes next most of all and I begin to shake uncontrollably.

The anesthesiologist arrives bearing the tools of the trade: the bagged IV fluid, rubber tubing, alcohol rubs, and needles. Yet while I abhor the task he must perform, at the same time I am strangely glad for his company. After he pricks my hand, I can feel the numbness taking affect, and he adeptly slides in the IV needle. I prefer not to watch. It doesn't hurt, but I can feel it, like a knitting needle being inserted slowly but painlessly under the skin. The anesthesiologist tapes it up all nice and neat like gift wrapping, and hooks the protruding hollow plastic connectors to the rubber hosing and IV bag. The coolness of the fluid crawls up my arm. When he injects a sedative through the tubing I can feel it creep through my bloodstream and overcome my senses.

The room begins to spin, and I am overtaken by a sensation akin to nausea. I quit trembling then, and quit caring about the state of my appendages. Yet I hold onto a tension the sedative is unable to ease. It doesn't matter how many times I've done this before. It doesn't get any easier and it's still scary.

When my surgeon finally arrives, I am glad to see him if only because the waiting is over. I can never resist tossing out a few of what I hope are witty remarks even in my current state as I am wheeled into the chill of the operating room. *Why does it have to be so bloody cold? Like a morgue.*

My last conscious thoughts compare the OR I am in to the museum replica in London's Science Museum. I intend to voice this to my doctor, but I am not sure the words ever emerge.

I awaken to the sound of rasping, and become dully aware that it is my own breath. When my vision clears, it is to see the huddled trio of my doctor and assisting surgeons peering down at me. I am told that there was some difficulty and that the breathing tube has to be reinserted. Before the thought of objection becomes concrete enough to express, I lose consciousness.

I awaken again to the awareness that my breathing is still labored, with the added sensation of a foreign object literally forcing back the walls of my throat, which have swollen up around it.

Saturday night, Sunday and Monday blend together such that any brief consciousness cannot be given a time label. I am aware that I am in intensive care, and that my mother is with me quite a bit of the time. Although I can see a clock I constantly ask what day it is. I have to be sure that precious days are not slipping away. I'm not sure how I asked, as I am obviously unable to speak.

Even during those first few days of heavy sedation, I maintain some cognition. I am well aware of the discomfort of the tubes, especially as sensation returns to areas initially desensitized by drugs and shock. Indeed, my hands are bound at first to prevent me ripping the intruding tubes from my face. The restraints annoy me almost more than the tubes. In one dream I am a corralled horse; a captive creature fighting. I awake, the tube silencing a scream of rage and my hands strain against their bindings. I am not one who takes easily to confinement.

I want those tubes out. This message is most common among my frantic scrawling and sign language which is my only form of communication. I do not believe I would have yanked those tubes out, although this conclusion is based exclusively on rational thoughts. The sensation of removing the tubes, especially with the force required if I were to take them in hand and tug, would stall the rational mind from such an effort. Yet in pain and under sedation, I am not always rational.

When I am awake and self-aware, getting my hands free becomes an obsession; a mind game to amuse myself and to deliberately defy my captors. I succeed once, twisting and pulling until my right hand is free. I lay my arm peacefully across my body and sleep in comfort. The nurse catches me innocently probing my face with my free hand. Having no mirror, touch is my most reliable sense. I feel the tubes, the swelling, and the bandages. But then my hand is snatched away and rebound.

If only the confinement and the necessity of tubes had been the worst of the experience, but there is more in store. I perceive that I am roughly handled and am unable to fight back in any way. In one instance, the nurses are manipulating me around the bed and one of them asks if I can roll over on my left side. I have a vague impression that I am not supposed to, so I shake my head violently "no." I have no other way to communicate this. "Sure you can," is what seems to me to be her callous reply, and over I am pushed. I cannot express the pain. It is as if all my insides are shifting and tearing. All I can do is lay there and bear it in silent agony and anger, assigning mental obscenities to the nurse responsible. Undoubtedly I express my distress in writing later.

For reasons I never know or never accept, the breathing tube has to be cleaned periodically. They send any visitors out of the room when performing this procedure. I now understand two sensations: suffocation and drowning. With no air in my lungs, and keep in mind I have no way to control air intake let alone hold my breath, the breathing tube is blocked off. Try it. Blow out all your air and seal your mouth and nose. Hold it. More, to the state of panic that inevitably follows. Add water to the vacuum- water which your lungs reject but cannot force out without violent spasms of attempted coughs and desperate sputtering. Add to this the violent quaking of a damaged abdomen, violated by fresh incisions which seem to tear at every movement.

By this time my veins have dried up. Those blood suckers are stubborn; jab after jab until the tears of frustration, intolerance, and pain stream down my face, yet they continue to jab until they somehow succeed.

During my five day stay in the Intensive Care Unit, I return to the operating room twice. The first is on Sunday, to remove a hematoma, or pooling of blood. They also have to release some of the skin on my neck because it cannot stretch enough on its own to accommodate the swelling. After so many previous procedures, my skin is tight and has limited expansion ability.

Persistent swelling and spiking fevers send me back to the OR on Tuesday. The omental flap, or transplanted fatty tissue, is removed. Though it seems to have good blood supply, parts are non-viable, as confirmed by a biopsy. Given my compromised condition, the surgeons elect to remove the flap entirely. I am wide awake, even cheerful for this one, though I can't imagine why I'd be so merry when I'm about to have the most crucial part of the surgery undone. Undoubtedly it is due to being alive, conscious and responsive, as well as to the information that my breathing tube would likely come out the following morning. Good news serves to dull or wash away unpleasantness. I remember having a conversation with the doctor. This must be a trick of memory because all I am able to do is write.

Daily pictures make sure that the spaghetti of tubing remains in good position, as well as track the comings and goings, while also revealing that all is well with my heart and lungs. At least something seems to be going right.

Tuesday is the first day I am allowed visitors aside from immediate family, and that is the day I find out that my surgery had lasted ten and a half hours, double the intended time. It didn't take nearly as long to be undone.

Wednesday morning the tube comes out. It feels like a snake slithering up my windpipe, enraging the raw sensitive tissue of my throat and nasal passages. The sensation is excruciating, like brushing an area where all your skin has been burned or rubbed off. My throat is swollen and sore, my voice weak and hoarse, but to the amazement of my ears I CAN SPEAK! With the spell of silence broken, I give my vocal cords plenty of exercise. However my voice remains raspy for the next several weeks.

Chapter Twenty Nine
With Great Resolve

For the first time in days I am hungry. I start on ice cubes, which are not the most delectable cuisine, yet the coolness is undeniably pleasant to my burning mouth and raw throat. I progress shortly to water, but it makes me nauseous in a most unpleasant manner, as an empty stomach has nothing to offer up.

Also, for the first time in days, I experience vertical motion. The unsteadiness is unavoidable, as weakened muscles refuse my weight and cannot respond to my head's demand for balance. But once I get it all worked out, mobility is exhilarating.

I am served flavor for breakfast on Thursday; a clear liquid diet, but a start. After all that time being fed through a needle, my stomach has to readjust to food. Consequently, though I am hungry, I have little appetite.

I move out of the intensive care unit that same day, and am settled into a room upstairs in the new plastic surgery ward. Aside from the luxuries of not having a catheter and being able to use tampons, the move means being unplugged from a myriad of wires, a step up in diet, and having a window and a mirror. Well, the mirror isn't a pleasant addition. It offers my first post-surgery look at myself, and I am a mess. My face protrudes in odd directions and I see for the first time the alteration in the skin of my left eye, literally sewn up on one side but all puffy and swollen. My face is discolored by bruising, iodine, stitches, dressings and dried blood. In fact, there is little that resembles normal skin. After a week of stress and no washing, my hair feels and behaves like matted straw and wire.

Wherever I go, the IV pole goes with me. I'd walk around even more, since my great resources of energy are gradually being restored, if the IV pole wasn't so cumbersome.

That night is a long one and filled with odd visions. The air conditioning is such that I either sweat or freeze. I wake up wet with sweat, then shiver as I try to air dry. My oddest vision is at first subconscious, because I am aware of it before I actually awaken enough to concentrate on the image. My IV pole stands silhouetted against the window, with its multi-hangars, single bag, and electronic box, looking almost like a person standing over me. It is not a comforting image; rather, a cold silent sentinel more like a scarecrow than a guardian angel.

I get little peaceful sleep that night, between the sweat and the icicles, but as I enjoy a quiet morning slumber I am interrupted by a 6 am doctor's call. He has only good news: my diet is to be upgraded, the IV is to come out, and I am to go home within the next couple of days.

As predicted, the elimination of the awkward IV pole facilitates my movement and I take to roaming the halls. A major step toward liberation.

Nothing is as blessed as running water. I can dip every part of my wretched, emaciated body under the warm flowing stream except my head. I bask in its healing powers, soaping away the days in bed until my strength gives out. A nurse takes me to a specially configured sink to wash my hair, ridding it of greasy stiffness and tangles of matted blood.

On Saturday, I am released from the hospital. Fresh air and freedom meet me on the sidewalk. But my ordeal is not yet over.

Post-discharge, the scar under my left cheek, which has been surgically reopened so many times now figures it knows what to do on its own, proceeds to reopen itself. At my first check-up, my doctor gives it nary a glance. I ignore the increasing ugliness of the wound, more likely out of stubborn denial rather than because of any rational thinking. I am determined that by sheer willpower I can make it all right. This is the second time stoicism gets the better of common sense, but it is my psyche's way of telling me I've had enough of doctors and hospitals. However, one day my mother panics at the sight of it and drags me in to see the doctor. I do not argue because deep inside I know she is probably correct and this incision really shouldn't be looking like that.

The following Tuesday sees my mother on an airplane back to Virginia and me in the doctor's office for clinical surgery with an opening that is doing a respectable imitation of the Grand Canyon. I am awake for this surgery, so I can feel all the pulling and tugging and cutting and stretching and stitching. My doctor has to cut the skin on my neck loose to be able to pull it over the gap. I rather enjoy knowing by *feel* every step of the procedure. Even with the IV drugs which are intended to relax me, I am still tense. But the chasm is successfully closed and in time it heals normally.

For the first time, I experience long-term pain as a result of what should have been a corrective procedure. As a result of the rather lengthy incision required to remove the failed omental flap, I suffer persistent abdominal pain. While not intense in nature, the twinges are fairly constant and do not completely subside for nearly a year. Since the abdominal muscles have been compromised and the area is tender, my martial arts studies are adversely affected for a time as well. To add insult to injury, this is pain with no gain since the transplanted flap didn't take and had to be removed. It feeds a growing resentment.

The bone graft into my cheek is successful, and there are no complications associated with the reshaping of the opening around my eye, so at least those parts of the procedure have gone as planned. However, there is no substitute for the muscles designed to hold things in place. The left eye opening remains different in shape from that of the right eye, so even this part of the procedure falls short of the desired result.

The ordeal leaves me with a deep-seated anger I cannot shake. The success of the previous two surgeries gave me optimism that my surgeon could make constructive changes, but with this procedure the reality of the medical limitations comes crashing in around me. It is not merely the notion that something we tried didn't work. Rather, it is the spectacular nature of that failure that causes me to call it all into question.

I don't blame my surgeon. Sometimes what works in theory goes awry in practical application and there are unintended consequences. In fact, I even go back to him and discuss what we might try next, but nothing my surgeon presents to me is enticing enough to want me to continue. I am becoming disenchanted.

My father suggests finding another surgeon, but that would be like starting over and I don't want to do that either. Besides, I'm not convinced anyone else can do any better. I'm gaining a broader understanding of my physical limitations. No active nerve means there is nothing to animate the muscle, so the paralysis remains, and the paralysis is the culprit behind the asymmetry.

I am not too keen on the idea of harvesting more pieces from elsewhere in my body for future transplants. These are what seem to cause the most complications and long term discomfort. In addition to facial scars, I have scars under each breast, down my belly, on my hip and a huge one down the inside of my left leg. My scars are measured in feet rather than inches and I'd rather not go for yardage.

The realization that I am fed up doesn't happen overnight. The physical and mental devastation from the most recent effort mean that I am in no hurry to jump back in the pool, even if I am testing the waters by making inquiries.

I am not afraid. Even though the unintended consequences nearly killed me, it is unlikely the next procedure would offer a repeat performance of that nightmare. But it does bring to mind cost, which could well be a pound of flesh lost to another failed transplant. Payment in scar tissue, payment in physical trauma and mental anguish, payment in pain and payment in recovery time, but to what end?

A face that children will still stare at.

Because no matter what we are able to accomplish, I will still look different. The degree of difference matters little.

I accept my incapacity with great resolve.

But acceptance doesn't automatically make everything better. It doesn't create impervious emotional armor, as much as I'd like it to.

Chapter Thirty
Expressions

I come home one day from the university and park on the street near my duplex. It is mid-afternoon of a gray day, and I labor with my pack of textbooks and proceed along the sidewalk toward home, done with the day's classes.

A woman and her son, who is probably around 7 years old, are coming out of the little dentist office next door right about the time I reach the path leading up to my door. I can see my cat Fizzbin waiting for me in the window and I smile, readying my house key.

I hear a child's voice yell after me.

"Retard!"

Alarmed, I turn to face my verbal attacker.

The mother gives me a furtive glance and shuffles the boy into a car, which is parked at the curb in front of me. All I can manage is a glare of hurt, surprise and anger. I toss the mother a glance, expecting a reprimand, but she remains silent. She avoids making eye contact with me. I can't seem to muster an appropriate reply of my own. My joy at returning home is crushed under this affront and all I can do is retreat to the solitude of my apartment and the comfort of my big orange cat. He is so glad to see me, oblivious of the slight I'd just received. I shouldn't really care about the cruel outburst of a misguided and socially maladapted child. But I do.

The comebacks come to mind too late, as I stew over the occurrence hours later.

The mother was probably embarrassed into silence. I would like to believe that mom at least had a discussion with Junior in the car on the way home regarding his rude behavior, but I suspect nothing meaningful was said. That being the case, I am appalled at the deficit in child-rearing skills that would allow such offensive behavior to go without correction. To ignore it is to encourage it. Even if she perceived me that way herself, it is nonetheless inexcusable.

I have no doubt that my appearance is the culprit. Never mind that I'm laden with college textbooks returning home from classes to the apartment that I occupy alone. This ill-mannered child has missed these other cues and reached his erroneous conclusion by assuming the face reflects the mind. If my face is imperfect, I must therefore be mentally incapacitated.

I met a woman with Down Syndrome several years ago. I am really glad that someone gave me a heads up that despite having the classic physical features associated with the condition, she exhibits what seems to be a normal IQ. I might otherwise have assumed that her Down Syndrome would be associated with inhibited mental development, which would have been unfair with this particular individual. Right or wrong, it is part of our social conditioning.

The human face, after all, is enormously important as a communication tool. I'm not referring to what we say, though my directness and occasional lack of forethought in what I utter has certainly been the source of great miscommunication. It's hard to walk away on a foot that is planted firmly in one's mouth. I refer instead to the expression and inflection of the face itself. The twitch of an eye, the hardening or softening of muscles, the shape of the lips forming a smile as it pushes the cheeks up, wrinkles the face and lights up the eyes. Like everyone else, I grew up reading other people's faces and learning which expressions are appropriate for which occasions. But in my case, only half the tools are working. I can only raise one eyebrow, narrow one eye, and can only flash a crooked smile. I do my best to imitate learned expressions that convey a particular meaning in our society, but I wonder if people get the message I intend to send. Sometimes their reaction is totally the opposite of what I expect, which leaves me confused and usually apologizing, baffled as to how they could have mistaken my intent.

It reminds me of the times I get passionate about a subject and my voice goes up, and people accuse me of yelling at them. I stare at them in shock. I'm not yelling *at* them. They are not the target, just the audience. It utterly amazes me that they can think it's about *them*. Then I become annoyed with them for being so sensitive and derailing the discussion.

In elementary school, a group of my peers once asked me to show facial expressions associated with different emotions.

"Show a happy face," someone said.

I smiled as genuinely as I could, though I didn't feel especially happy. They commented and one or two of them laughed. I was not hurt or insulted by their amusement. I enjoyed the attention, and was a little impressed that they showed what seemed to be genuine, innocent curiosity. Whatever the intention, I didn't feel like I was being ridiculed or mocked. I've always enjoyed making people laugh, with the only exception being a deliberate affront.

"Now sad," another said. My face changed as best it could.

"Ok, angry!"

I concentrated on that emotion, trying to make it happen.

"I didn't see any change," someone remarks.

"Well, since I'm not actually angry I can only pretend," I defended.

Yet I am disturbed by this. If people still have trouble distinguishing my expression of sadness from that of anger, this could definitely lead to some misinterpretations. Are some signals completely missed because they are incomprehensible? If so, it could be said that my face speaks a different language, and if that language is unique to itself, no one else can be expected to comprehend it. That puts me in an awkward and frustrating position. I believe I am conveying one emotion, but it is being read as another. Worse yet, if my face is unreadable, an observer might assume that there is nothing behind it. After all, a blank stare generally relays total incomprehension.

I am often told by friends that once they get to know me, they don't notice my face anymore. Perhaps part of what they really mean is that they've learned its language.

Regardless of the conclusions the child outside the dentist office came to, I ponder what possessed him to shout out that incorrect yet hurtful label. Could it be that it is human nature to chastise and separate out those who are different? I certainly have felt like an outcast, finding solace and companionship amongst other misfits. Perhaps his is learned behavior, stemming from the attitude of the family. Or it could be as simple as lack of exposure. If one does not interact with people who are "different," one has no way to learn to relate to them. I wasn't raised around anyone else with a physical disability. I catch myself noticing other people who have a physical difference, and all I have to go on is how I prefer to have people interact with me.

When I am nervous or afraid, sometimes it manifests as impatience or anger. I worry that if children are afraid of those of us who are physically flawed, they are in danger of growing up bigoted and intolerant as a way to mask their own insecurity. They may lash out in the form of bullying, thus creating a false sense of superiority, which is what I believe the unruly child did when he encountered me.

Perhaps this redefines the value of my brief involvement with the Boys and Girls Club. I work for a time as an on-call substitute staff person, not only exposing children of varying ages to someone who has an imperfect face, but who is also an authority figure. If a child asks me about my face, I answer as simply, kindly and honestly as possible. I try to conduct myself fairly and indeed in this respect I am no different from any other staff member. My appearance may be more memorable, but otherwise I emphasize that I am no different from anyone else.

Back in high school, some of my school friends take on a punk or Goth look, adding purple, yellow, green, or burgundy tints to hair which had already been dyed black. They have multiple ear piercings, before the days when it becomes the norm to find the most painful places on one's body to impale. They wear black and shop at second hand clothing stores for the oddest styles possible. Except for having an affinity for wearing black, I do not partake in their forms of self-expression.

"How would you describe the way I dress?" I ask Murray. I can think of no category so I am genuinely curious.

"I would call it conservative," is his reply.

"Huh." A statement, not a question.

Jeans, T-shirts, turtlenecks, sweatshirts, hoodies, athletic shoes; that is my standard fare and what makes me comfortable. Any time I've departed from my nondescript attire, I have an internal sense of mistaken identity, like a leopard airbrushing over my spots with tawny paint. A costume can be fun, but an attempt at creating a false image can backfire.

I tend not to show much skin or wear tight clothing, though I have been told on occasion that doing so would flatter me. My upbringing has not been one of flaunting my body, no matter how well-developed and shapely it might be. Indeed, I might be able to use it to distract people from my face, but that is not the type of attention I seek.

I rarely put on make-up, with one notable exception: when my eyebrows fall prey to the trichotillomania. It isn't so much that I rebel against the cosmetic industry. Rather, I feel it's a waste of time. I have better things to do than stand before a mirror smearing goo on my face. I am blessed with a favorable complexion, but let's be honest. It's not like make-up is going to hide the blemishes and no amount of enhancement will detract from my most prominent facial features.

I've never been seriously tempted by tattoo art either. I've been poked by enough needles in my time that having a tattoo done completely loses any appeal. I also have reservations regarding the permanence of the image. I prefer more temporary forms of self-expression, like t-shirts, for example.

Chapter Thirty One
The Kindness of Strangers

In early 1988, I am approaching graduation. Adrian has been commissioned to write a textbook for his popular Cinema class at the University. A prominent publishing company out of the Midwest has counted the number of students who take his most popular class each term and has determined that there is an opportunity here to make some money. Adrian, meanwhile, could care less whether the publishing company makes any money or not.

As Adrian toils away, he tasks me with finding, acquiring, and obtaining permission to publish stills from the various films he discusses in the text of his opus. My employment with the Media Services Center finds me often in the projection booth for Adrian's classes so I am quite familiar with the films he uses. I get paid to watch these films, over and over. He does vary the films from term to term, but there are quite a few constants.

Unwilling and unable to make the trip himself, Adrian manages to convince the publisher to send me to Los Angeles to research and obtain cinematic stills at the Margaret Herrick Library at the Academy of Motion Picture Arts and Sciences. Housed here are millions of production stills, including many from little-known or largely forgotten cinematic works. These are exactly the types of films Adrian subjects his students to.

Los Angeles! I am lured by Hollywood's luster, especially since I have aspirations of working in the film industry. I figure my best shot is through my writing, though I'd rather be a film director. Any excuse to visit LA is a thrilling proposal.

As soon as I determine that the trip is a "go" and have my dates figured out, I write letters to my two potential show business contacts to determine if they are willing and available to meet with me.

One is writer/producer Allan Burns, with whom I've now been corresponding for approximately the last 10 years. He agrees to meet and gives me his contact information so I can let him know when I am actually in town so we can set up a meeting. I am thrilled beyond imagination, but nervous as well.

The other is the highly successful writer/producer Stephen Cannell. In his letter to me six years previous, Mr. Cannell offered to meet with me "if I am ever in Los Angeles." I contact his office to take him up on the offer. Regrettably, he is to be out of town during my visit (on his yacht writing I'm told), so I am set up with an associate. I am to contact her when I get to town to set up the meeting time.

This gives my trip a whole new dimension. I am presented with an opportunity to sell my ability and show off my talent. But am I ready for this? I haven't written anything notable since high school. *But I can't take that material. It is too old, and reads like it was written by the immature teenager that I was.*

I settle instead on an adaptation I made of one of Adrian's stories, which I plan to produce as a student movie. The piece is cynical and not my original work, plus our styles and areas of thematic expertise are very different. However, it is available, current, and I have nothing original to offer. I am a writer who has not been writing.

When the day finally arrives, I depart SeaTac on a morning flight, so have plenty of time left in the day when I arrive at LAX.

I've arranged a rental car and the pick-up goes without a hitch, which is good because this is my first time ever renting a car. For a young driver, Los Angeles is an education. All the stories you hear about California drivers are true, but I shouldn't ridicule. As an inexperienced driver unfamiliar with the area, I fit right in.

The Margaret Herrick Library is housed on Wilshire Boulevard in Beverly Hills and I find it with minimal trouble. Beverly Hills is an erection in the surrounding skyline, a hard ostentatious cluster of taller office buildings jutting out amidst a much flatter array of dwellings and complexes. I enter the building armed with a catalogue of Adrian's oft-used but obscure and bizarre film titles including *Eraserhead, Zardoz, Interiors* and *Brazil*. In typical library fashion, this one has shelves of books with a row of reading tables down the center. However, I proceed to the back of the room where a clerk sits behind a counter in front of another sizable room, awaiting photo requests. I give the clerk the titles I need, and she pulls the files for me to peruse at one of the tables. With over 7 million stills in the Library's collection, I am bound to find most of what I need. I opt to photocopy anything potentially interesting so that Adrian can make the final selection himself. As I settle at a table to examine a handful of files, I find myself sitting near a middle aged woman with hair colored faintly red.

I'm so happy and excited to be here that I greet her amiably and we strike up polite conversation. I tell her about my photo research project, and learn that she is a freelance reporter digging up photos for an article she's writing. I introduce myself and she tells me her name is Lena.

"You wouldn't happen to be able to recommend a good place to stay, would you?" I finally ask. "Not too expensive. I'm a poor college student."

"Didn't you set anything up in advance?"

"No. I figured something would work out. There has to be lots of places."

I've arranged places to stay with former university students for part of my trip, but fell short on finding somewhere for the first couple of nights. I got so used to winging it in Great Britain, I figured I could do so here as well.

Lena ponders a moment.

"How long do you need to stay?" she inquires.

"Just a couple of nights," I reply. "I'll be staying with some people I know after that."

"You can stay with me," she says quickly.

I pick my jaw up off the table.

"Are you serious? I mean, I appreciate the offer, but are you sure?" I reply incredulously.

"Sure," she says. She writes down her information along with directions to her place and hands it to me. She sets an arrival time, then leaves to take care of other business. I can't believe my luck, and her unexpected trust. She is not the only one taking a risk, but it hardly occurs to me not to return that trust.

I'm not the typical archetype who gravitates to LA. Is Lena such a good judge of character that she can tell that I am sincere in my words and of good integrity? Or do I just not fit the profile of a serial killer? Maybe I have an honest face. But I decide not to look a gift horse in the mouth.

I kill time driving around and familiarizing myself with the area. I venture up La Brea, past the tar pits and along Hollywood Boulevard. I spot the famous landmarks such as the Walk of Fame and Mann's Chinese Theater and ogle them as I drive past. I am surprised at how close everything is. Burbank, Studio City, Culver City; all these famous studio suburbs seem just blocks away from each other with little separation between them. Neighborhoods and business districts blend together so that only signs distinguish one from another.

As I reach the lesser developed end of Hollywood Boulevard, I stumble headlong into one of my destinations: the many-storied glass paneled building with the letters in familiar font printed across the top: *Stephen J. Cannell Productions*. I am told that when the highly successful *A-Team* was sold into syndication, the revenue funded this brand new building, hence nicknaming it "the house that A-Team built." I am in awe and a wave of excitement and anticipation passes through me. What's more, I can probably even find it again.

I proceed onward to Sunset Boulevard, and turn right for the ascent toward Lena's house. And what an ascent it is. I pass a street vendor selling maps to the stars' homes. I wonder if Lena has any notable neighbors. As I climb higher on the twisting turning pavement which is more like a series of ramps than a road, the Bob Seger tune *Hollywood Nights* keeps playing in my head, especially the line about "those Hollywood hills." It is getting dark, and there are times I can see past the houses and through the trees and bushes to the lights below. I find Lena's little house nestled inside a curve. It is a tiny cottage compared to the neighboring multi-storey homes, some of which might qualify as mansions. Whatever view it may have once had is now blocked by more expensive real estate hugging the hillside across the narrow street. But it has a cozy, non-threatening feel. I park where she has instructed, grab my suitcase, and knock timidly on the door.

Lena answers warmly, bifocals adorning her face.

"Come in," she greets.

"Your directions were excellent. I had no trouble finding the place. What a lovely little house you have! And a very fancy neighborhood!"

"Thank you," she says, showing me in. "My family bought this house 50 years ago for about $20,000. Of course the values have skyrocketed since then. We were grandfathered in on the old property tax system or else the taxes would be so high I wouldn't be able to afford to live here."

"Wow, good investment."

I amuse myself while she works on an article.

There isn't too much else to say about Lena, except that we get along well. We go on walks together around the neighborhood and chat pleasantly. She is devoted to her two little dogs and she is incredibly kind and generous to me. I learn that a close relative is one of the founders of a major studio, but was effectively cut out of the business so that others made all the money from it. Lena is a reporter of modest success and well received by Hollywood's older set of famed personalities. For example, she did the last-ever interview with Fred Astaire, was on set for the last day of shooting on the TV series M*A*S*H, and Bob Hope's wife Delores is considered a friend.

She became a friend to me when I needed one, even though I wasn't really looking, and trusted me in a city where trust is a rare commodity.

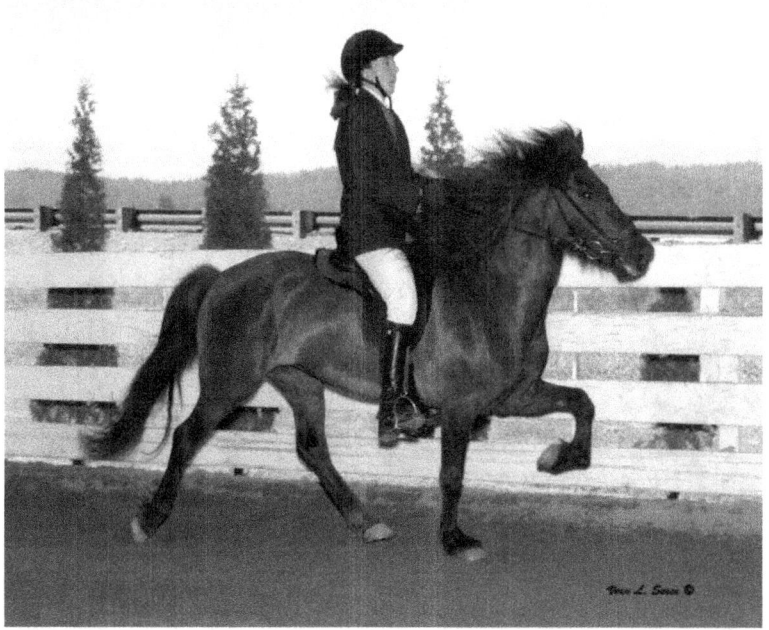

Me riding Askja, the talented mare I imported from Iceland in 2001.
Reprinted with permission from Vern L. Serex Enterprises ©2002.

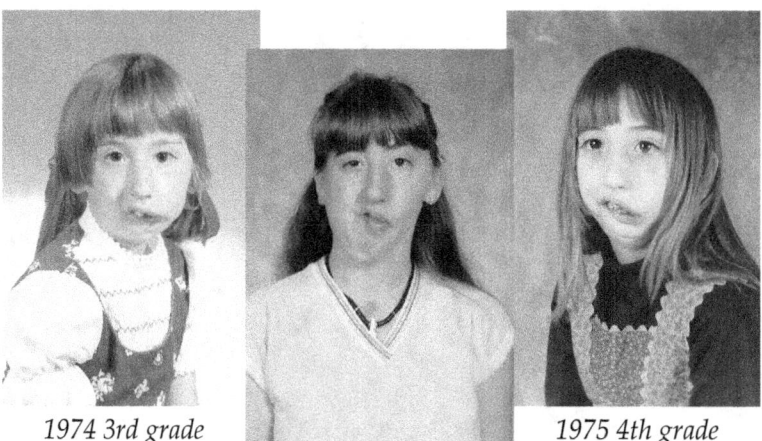

1974 3rd grade photo, age 8.

1982 11th grade photo, age 16.

1975 4th grade photo, age 9.

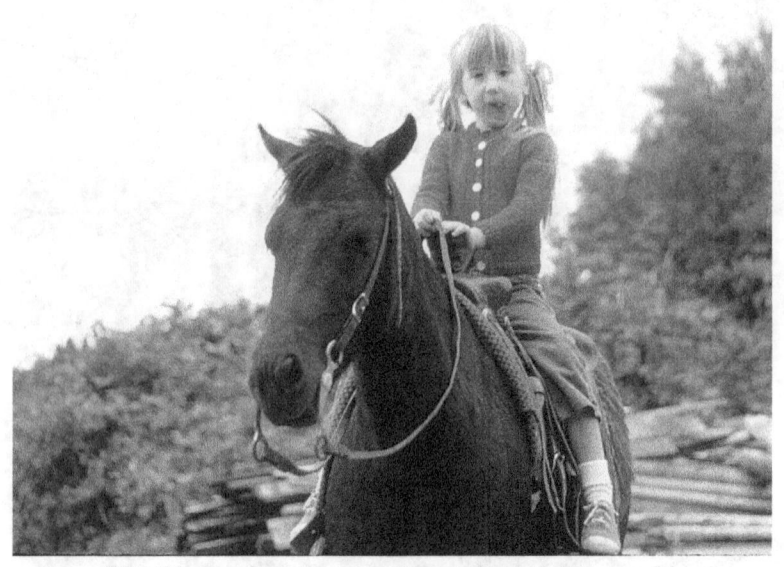

Possibly my first time on a horse. I was 3-5 years old.

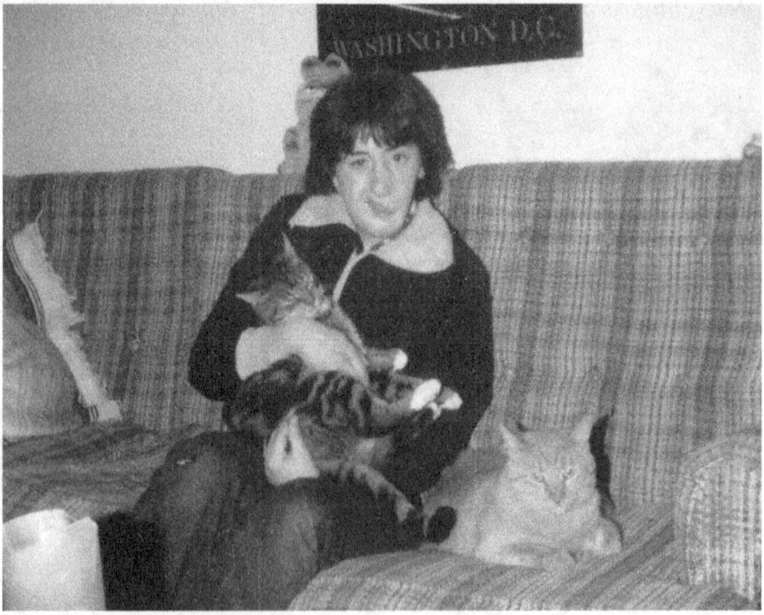

In my own apartment at college with Motley (in my arms) and Fizzbin, 1987 after my final facial surgery.

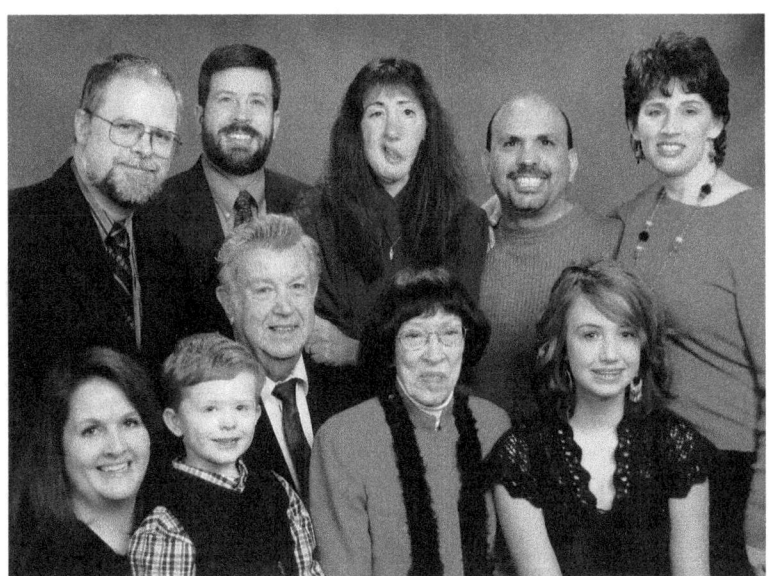

Family portrait taken in 2007 for my parents' 50th anniversary.
Reprinted with permission.

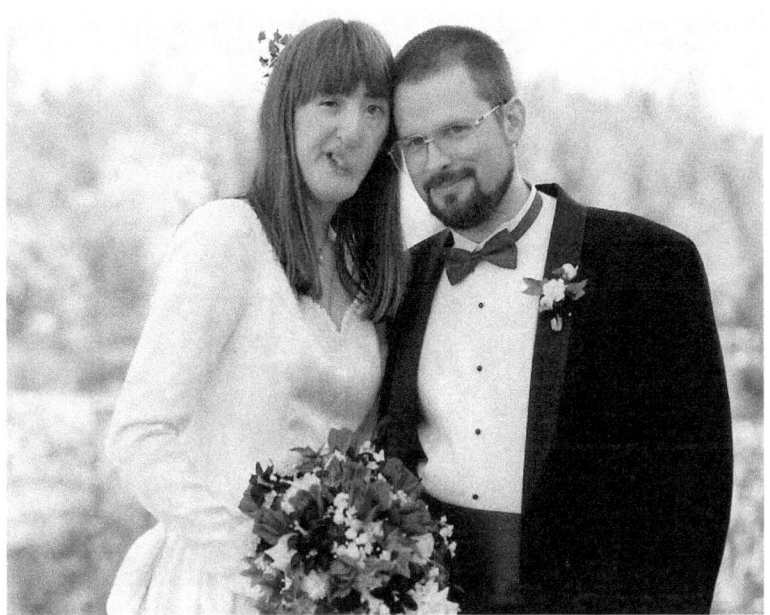

The bride and groom, September 23, 1995.

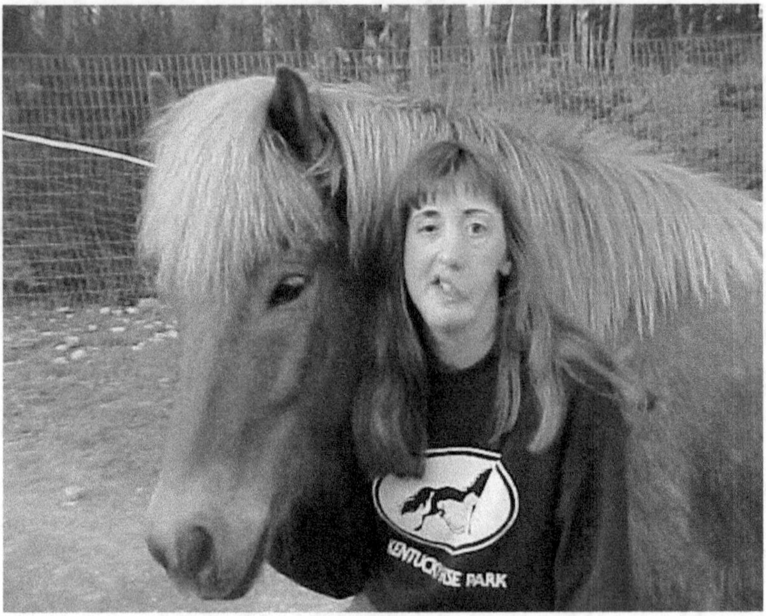

Me and Rísi, my first Icelandic horse. 1997

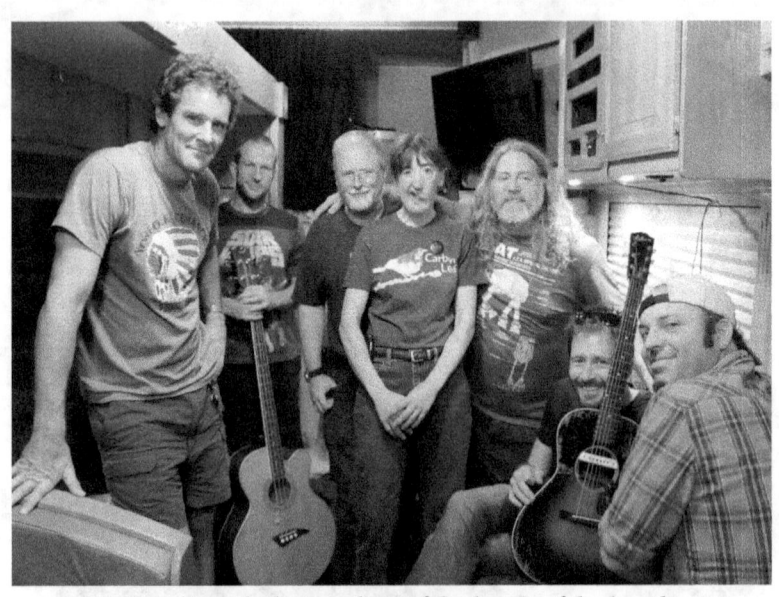

Ian and I with the members of Carbon Leaf during the fall tour of 2015.

Chapter Thirty Two
Presentation

During my time staying with Lena, I finalize my meeting times with Allan and with Stephen Cannell's associate. I also complete my work at the Margaret Herrick Library, collecting a stack of photocopies to take back with me along with information on how to order prints once our selections are made.

I move on to the residence of a young couple I know from the university, graduates from the Theater Department. They are renting a house about two blocks from one of the major studios which has high imposing solid walls stretching for blocks. The husband tells me that sometimes the streets are closed so they can film in the nearby neighborhoods.

I am to see Allan first. MTM Studios, 4024 Radford Ave, Studio City. How familiar that address looks. How excited it made me to read it on the return envelope of a letter or package. Now I am to have my first inside look at a major production studio.

My stomach has butterflies as I nervously drive up to the gate of MTM Studios and stop at the guard house.

"I'm here for a meeting with Allan Burns," I state.

"Name?"

"Oh, right. Dawn Daugherty."

He checks a piece of paper.

"Ok," he responds.

He offers directions to the building where Allan's office is. I feel a sense of importance as I pass through that gate. I am expected, and I am welcome.

However nervous I was driving in, I am threefold that as I approach his office. The butterflies are doing aerial maneuvers in my stomach. I clutch my bundle of material.

He smiles and greets me warmly as I enter his open office. His Emmy awards and other statuettes are proudly but tastefully displayed on shelves. It is a spacious office, but not gaudy or overbearing.

I realize that he has never seen a photo of me. My appearance must be a complete surprise to him, but he doesn't show it. I have make-up on, mostly to cover up zits, diffuse the facial scars and even out my complexion.

"We finally meet," he says. "What's it been, 10 years?"

"Yeah, something like that," I reply. He has done his best to put me at ease but I am still tense.

He queries me politely about my trip so far. I tell him about the photographic research and share that my next meeting is with an associate of Mr. Cannell. I thank him again for helping to facilitate that.

He notices my folder.

"Did you bring something for me to look at?" he asks.

"Yeah, if you want to. It's actually just an adaptation I made of a friend's work. So it really isn't mine. But I haven't been writing much lately. Too busy with college. Still, it's what I have."

I hand it over to him. I try to sit quietly and patiently as he glances over it.

"You really ought to be doing your own work," Allan finally says. "You showed a lot of potential."

"I have a problem with ideas," I reply honestly.

"This doesn't flow very well. The characters have no depth. There's no one to be sympathetic with."

He continues on. Though he is gentle with his criticism, it is obvious that he is unimpressed with the material. I have disappointed him. My heart sinks. I feel about 3 feet tall. My mind is reeling. *What have I done?*

He wraps up our session by announcing that he has a lunch meeting to attend.

"Is it OK if I walk around a bit?" I ask quietly.

"Sure," he replies. "I don't think there's much going on today. Just a rehearsal for a new show that Mary is doing. You could probably drop in on that."

"OK. Thanks. That sounds interesting." I am much more subdued.

We shake hands and part company. I am unsure if I will have any future correspondence. He didn't exactly tell me off, but didn't embrace me with encouragement either.

Still with heavy heart, I return to my car, dropping off the fateful folder and grab instead my still camera. I wander off toward the studios.

The place really is quiet. Not much activity at all that I can see on the vast grounds. No hustle and bustle that one might expect from a studio lot. Not even any cars moving about. The rehearsal for Mary Tyler Moore's new show, airing under the title "Annie McGuire" is easy enough to find since it is the only place with any sign of life. I walk into the area. They are actively rehearsing so I hang back out of the way. I've done enough theater work to understand the rehearsal process. The set is lit only with working lights, and there are no cameras. The plot involves a man in a wheelchair interacting with Mary's character. I get the impression the man's character is unemployed and bitter, possibly a veteran. The set is sparsely furnished, intending to represent the man's house. I spot an older Breyer horse model on one of the set pieces. This lifts my spirits slightly.

Though I successfully do not interfere, I fail at being inconspicuous. With so few people about and with me so obviously a stranger, the cast members who are not actively rehearsing are curious about my presence.

At a table far removed from the rehearsal, I sit and chat with the actors. I explain about my meeting with Allan. I'm sure my disappointment is obvious. Mary walks in. I stand up at the entry of a legend. She approaches me.

"Are you the documenting photographer?" she asks.

I glance down at the camera still strapped to my person. It has not left its protective case.

"Uh, no," I stumble, trying not to be star-struck in her presence. "I just came from a meeting with Allan Burns. We'd been corresponding for a number of years. I'm hoping to be a writer."

"Oh. And your name is?"

"Dawn. Sorry."

We shake hands.

"Mary," she responds. As if I didn't know. "Allan is wonderful, isn't he?"

"Yes, he is. I am very grateful that he was kind enough to meet with me."

"So how did your meeting go?" she asks.

"Not too well," the sinking feeling sets in again. "I don't think he was very impressed with the material I brought. Rightfully so. I mean, he was really nice about it. But I don't think he thought it was very good."

"Ah. Well, have a look around."

"Thanks. Nice meeting you." I reply.

I don't stay much longer. Things become active again and people become involved with their work. Rehearsals are not exciting to watch, even in Hollywood.

If Allan didn't like my material, what could I expect from Stephen Cannell's associate?

Not much, as it turns out. The meeting was amiable enough,

made more pleasant by the fact that the woman I met with was British. She is polite, but I have nothing with which to truly impress her. She, too, asks me how my meeting with Allan went, and I don't know any better than to be honest about it. My personality is not charming enough to win her over and having never seen any evidence of my writing ability she really has no investment in this meeting other than her boss asked her to do it. I leave the script with her, but hear nothing more.

I like to believe that if I'd actually met with Mr. Cannell things might have gone differently. I tend to be more at ease with men, even ones with a certain celebrity. He and I both have had challenges to overcome, he with dyslexia and I, my face. This commonality might have given us a certain rapport that I was unable to have with his associate. But of course this does not change the fact that the material I had with me was uninspiring and not my own.

I may well have been better off not bringing any of my work with me, and leaving it as a "getting acquainted" session. Now an adult, I have lost the immunity and allowance for making mistakes that being a "kid" originally gave me.

The rest of my trip is spent as a tourist, first on Hollywood Boulevard, then at Disneyland and Universal Studios.

My trip is successful in that the original purpose has been fulfilled. When I return to Washington, I turn over to Adrian a stack of photocopies. He chooses the ones he wants, and I set about obtaining permission to publish them. I correspond with Lena for a number of years, even visiting her again before finally losing touch.

In another respect, my trip is an utter and complete failure. Our lives are full of the "could-have-beens" and "what ifs." A different outcome might have set my life on a totally different path. I do my best to retain hope that not all is lost.

Not long after I return home, I am told second hand that something has gone horribly wrong with my relationship with Allan. I am given no specifics, but I am left with the impression it may have been something a cast member from the set had relayed to him. I don't remember saying anything terrible, but I'm sure my demeanor belied my disappointment in letting him down. I immediately send Allan a letter thanking him for meeting with me and apologizing for anything I might have said that was interpreted badly, but I never hear from him again. I had not proven myself worthy of his continued time and attention, or I had somehow offended him beyond repair. I will have to make my way without his help, but it is a disappointment and a loss I have never quite recovered from.

My appearance gives me an opportunity to make an impression, but what sort of impression is up to what's inside of me. First impressions can be difficult to overcome. If the impression I make is positive and good, it is long lasting and I am unforgettable. But likewise if I fail to impress then my unforgettable-ness becomes a liability. Oh, yes, I will be remembered, but for all the wrong reasons.

The lesson learned is this: If you aspire toward a certain goal, you need to be continually working toward that goal. *If you want to be a writer, write.* I was not writing. Pure and simple. I was not developing my craft or utilizing my talent. The piece I offered did not reflect what I am capable of when I put my mind, heart and soul into my writing. I blew this opportunity as surely as if I'd pulled out a gun, aimed it at my foot, and pulled the trigger.

My physical uniqueness may help make me memorable, but it is what I have to offer as a human being that makes the lasting impression. What I presented that day of myself and my work was unremarkable.

Chapter Thirty Three
Burning Candles and Getting Burned

I do have various writing projects going, but they amount to little more than exercises. While I may not be writing producible or publishable material, I am keeping plenty busy.

I keep attaching myself to various theatrical productions. I now have more friends in the Theater Department thanks to my European travels, and my prior experience makes me more desirable on crew. I have the pleasure of working as property master and assistant stage manager to Michelle on a production directed by my former acting instructor. That's right, the one who gave me a "C" in his acting class. This production wins an award and we take it on the road to the next level of competition. Though it fails to go any further, I am nonetheless very pleased to be a part of a high quality show.

Theater classes are seldom held at 8 AM, probably because most of the instructional staff is also involved in these various productions. Rehearsals and most performances are in the evenings and often run late, so no one wants to get up for an early class.

However, my primary major isn't Theater. It is Visual Communications, and those instructors have no qualms at all about holding classes at 8 am. Yet somehow even after late night rehearsals or performances, I manage to stumble to class. I certainly understand the concept of burning the candle at both ends.

I don't quite have what I need to graduate in four years. By spring of 1988 I am close, but I need one or two more vital classes for my Bachelor of Science degree, which thankfully are offered fall quarter. If I stay a little longer, I'll complete the class and credit requirements for a Bachelor of Arts in Theater as well. In the summer of '88 I decide to stay in town and sign up for the Summerstock program. This is a series of plays produced over the summer, and is considered credited coursework. Though I dropped out of light design class because it was way over my head, I still have an interest in lighting, and I want nothing more than to learn to run the light board during a production. Prior to enlisting in the program, I ask the department head if this can be arranged, and he assures me that it can. But apparently he is like a politician or an enlistment officer, telling people what they want to hear even if he is unable to back up his promises.

As each show comes and goes, I am not asked nor offered to have anything to do with running the light board. For most of the summer, I sit passively back in my role as technical lackey. Finally, as we are running out of shows, I bring it up to the Maker of the Promise and he informs me that the grad students have priority in that position so that opportunity will not be offered me. I subsequently label the experience *Summerstock of my Discontent*, and learn an important lesson about making sure that agreements are put in writing.

For my Visual Communications major, I have to provide a senior project. I decide to produce the adaptation I'd done of Adrian's story as a movie, even though the script let me down during my Los Angeles visit. I figure I might as well get some use out of it, and I have no better options.

I take on many of the production roles singlehandedly. I don't have much prior experience doing this, so I wing it. I decide to do all the camera work myself, and for budget reasons I have little choice but to use home-consumer VHS cameras. I recruit actors from the Theater Department and am able to hand-pick most of them. The majority say yes without hesitation. Adrian is popular in the department and the students are happy to help bring one of his works to life. Also, being in a video movie is a departure from stage work and many would like to add such experience to their acting resume.

It feels good to head up a team of talented people who are enthusiastic about working with me on this project. I love being in charge, though I confess to not always taking charge. I can be indecisive sometimes, but this allowed my cast and crew to have input even if they may sometimes lose patience.

The story, titled *Too Stupid to Live*, is a black comedy centering around a factory worker whose hobby is making bombs, and as events seem to turn more and more against him (a bad day taken to extremes), his solution is to blow everything up as he descends into madness.

I may have my weak points in terms of leadership, but one thing I can do is organize and form a schedule. I would have made a good production manager had I set my sights in that direction.

Locations are a particular challenge, but my student status goes a long way toward getting me what I need. An acquaintance puts me in touch with a property owner who gives us access to an empty building on the waterfront and this becomes the factory where the main character works. One of the guys I work with in Media Services lets us use the exterior of his house as the main character's house. I am able to "borrow" a police car and a tow truck. My car is being used as the main character's car, and it gets wrecked in the movie. I don't show the accident of course, but will imply it using sound effects. After searching several junkyards, I am able to find a smashed up car which looks enough like mine to be its double, which the main character then visits to retrieve something he needs.

At the local hospital, we run into a bit of a problem. We are allowed a room and set up our main character in the bed with a hospital gown. We bandage him up, hang an IV bag on a stand next to the bed, and tape tubes to his hand for added realism. Even without needles the mock-up makes me wince. This scene takes place after the car accident, and our anti-hero is in a coma, so the actor's job is to lie still during the entire scene. His smothering and usually disapproving mother is played by a boisterous woman with excellent vocal projection.

"My poor son!" she wails. "Why is he just lying there? Can't anyone *do* anything?"

She continues her lines which follow the same vein. A floor nurse interrupts our rehearsal.

"Um, I understand you're shooting a student movie," she says gently. "But I need to ask you to keep it down. You're upsetting some of the patients."

I don't know whether to be mortified that we're causing a disruption after we've been generously allowed to use the space, to laugh and be proud because my actress is doing such an effective portrayal, or to be disgruntled because I won't be able to capture the full effect of her performance.

Of course I have to respect the hospital's wishes and direct my cast accordingly. "Mom" manages a loud whisper with perfect tone and inflection, thus pulling off the scene despite our limitations.

Except for the hospital gown and a police uniform which we are able to borrow, the actors provide their own costumes and clothing. I have a tiny budget sequestered from the Theater Department so can buy materials so I can make some of the props, including the cartoon style detonator for the "big" bomb at the end. I have to chase down sound effects, and Sean, Michelle's boyfriend, comes to the rescue by recording original music.

One of the Video Services employees is assigned as my editor and we master on ¾" videotape. Audio tracks are limited and we have to premix some stuff to get everything on there. After many hours in the edit room, we get it done. The technical quality isn't stellar because we had to shoot on VHS and because the editing equipment is old. It doesn't quite end up movie length- an hour, maybe a little longer, but it's plenty long enough.

It does not turn out brilliantly. In fact some of the actors are justifiably disappointed in the final cut. But it is my first attempt at such an endeavor and I realize afterward that I have little feel for pacing as many of the scenes go on way too long.

I receive an "A" on the project from the Technology Department, but more in recognition of effort rather than for being the next Steven Spielberg.

"It has to be the most ambitious project I've seen done," says the technology department head. This makes me feel good, despite recognizing the movie's shortcomings. And my own, for that matter.

I hope the people working with me had as much fun as I did. As someone who tends to be result oriented, this is one activity in which I can sincerely say I loved the process more than the end result.

At my karate school, I test for and am awarded a first degree black belt. I am told that this achievement signifies the beginning of learning, but for me, it proves to be the beginning of the end. Once I move away from my support system and am unable to find a replacement dojo close to where I live, I lose my motivation. I am proud of my achievement and still have regrets that I was unable to continue, but have little choice but to let it go and move on.

I walk through graduation at the end of fall quarter of 1988, having received all the credits I need to complete my Bachelor of Science in Visual Communications. I graduate cum laude. I stay on for two more quarters to complete my Bachelor of Arts in Theater. When I put in for that certificate, however, I am in for a rude shock.

Apparently, once you graduate, in order to earn a second degree you need to have a certain number of credits over and above what you had when you graduated. Do any of my advisors tell me this? *No.* In all fairness, it's some obscure rule that probably appears in microscopic print somewhere on page 647 of a thousand-page document. Had I waited and not walked through graduation after fall term, I could have graduated with two fully recognized degrees in the spring with no trouble at all.

I schedule a meeting with the president of the University to plead my case, but to no avail. He questions the policy, but does not offer any exceptions.

"Why are we keeping advanced students longer by insisting on more credits when we are turning away freshmen because we are too full?" he demands of the board of directors. "Isn't the idea to graduate people and move them along?"

"It's just a piece of paper," a University representative tells me helpfully. "It doesn't change the fact that you earned the credits and completed the requirements."

I try to take comfort in that, but when you graduate from college and enter the world of job-seeking, that piece of paper is one of the few tangible things you have. I cannot help but feel that there is a fundamental unfairness to this. I earned both degrees therefore I should be recognized for them both. But I've been there 5 years and that is enough of my life and enough of my parents' money spent. Besides, I've run out of course material.

I consider it a positive that it isn't the other way around. A Bachelor of Science in Visual Communications does have a more impressive ring to it than a Bachelor of Arts in Theater, especially when you are applying for jobs relating to video production.

Then again, neither makes a whit of difference when you are applying at Dairy Queen, which is to become my first job after returning home from college.

Chapter Thirty Four
But I'm not...

What is the one line that every college graduate should know?
Dramatic pause.
"Would you like fries with that?"

My dad knows the owner of a local Dairy Queen via the Lions Club, and through this connection I am able to get a job there. This owner has a policy of hiring people with disabilities, so it doesn't matter to him if the front counter isn't lined with pretty faces. I am self-conscious about being on public display, yet at the same time I am relieved that my employer doesn't feel that I need to be hidden away in the kitchen. The customers don't seem to treat me any differently or else I am too busy to notice.

I don't mind the work and get along well with most of the staff, but I soon discover that working in fast food is not my forté. I get frazzled under pressure and I don't always get the orders right. As a perfectionist who wants to excel at everything, this irks me. However, at least I can accurately count change.

In the meantime, through another connection of my father's, I find myself lined up for a volunteer position at the nearby Naval Undersea Warfare Engineering Station. My dad retired from here, and both my brother and sister are currently employed here. Apparently the facility is in the process of putting together a small video production department in conjunction with still photography. Operated by the Navy, it primarily employs civilians. However, a hiring freeze prevents any direct hiring with two notable exceptions: ex-military and people who come in through programs like the one they expect me to qualify for.

My resume isn't bad for being fresh out of college. As well as the Media Services job, I've done a couple of internships including one at an oil refinery where I'd single-handedly produced training videos. There I'd gained experience working in an industrial setting, feeling at home around noisy dirty machinery and wearing safety gear while I worked. So I have the type of education and experience the Navy is looking for.

Yet to qualify for this volunteer program, I have to be certified as disabled by Washington State's Department of Vocational Rehabilitation (DVR).

Wait…what? Disabled?

I may not have a pretty face, but I've never considered myself to be disabled. In fact, I feel awkward that I'm even being considered for this program. However, I want the position, and my potential co-workers who became employed via the same program believe that I will qualify and are very encouraging. Jobs in video production are difficult to come by, especially outside of a large city. If the volunteer position turns into a paid position, I'll have a good salary plus benefits working in a very competitive field. I decide to swallow my pride and treat it as a means to an end.

I do have to meet certain criteria. DVR services are available to anyone who has a physical, mental, cognitive or sensory disability that makes it difficult to work in a job that matches their skills, interests and potential, or that may cause a potential employer to discriminate against them. I haven't really thought about my appearance as a barrier to getting a job, but it is conceivable that an employer might discriminate against me for this reason. Since my disability is openly visible rather than hidden, I don't need a physical nor do I need to submit documentation of my medical history.

Having a position waiting, even if it is a volunteer position, is a definite plus. The application seems more of a formality, though I do have to be a little creative.

"So how does your disability limit your ability to perform this type of work?" the counselor asks.

"Well, I can't do my own voice-overs and I am unable to be used as on-screen talent," I reply lamely. As in theatrical production, I am limited in my performance capabilities, but it's hard to sound convincing because this is stuff I don't really need to do. For scripting, shooting, directing and editing, which would be my primary tasks, I am fully capable. I worry that they will reject me for being too "able." However, my interview and application are sufficient and I am accepted into the program.

My certification comes through In December of 1989. January 22, 1990 is my first day as a volunteer. After two short months, a paid position is created for me and by the end of March I am gainfully employed as an Audio Visual Production Specialist.

While delighted at this career opportunity, I am also humbled by the notion that a government agency considers me disabled when I've never previously viewed myself in that way. I take small comfort in being told that requirements for disability benefits on the federal level are much more stringent and I would likely not qualify. Fine with me.

Yet I used the system to advance my career, which gives me a degree of guilt. Does this mean I can be disabled when convenient? Or am I disabled only when others perceive me as such?

In July of 2006, I attend an Indigo Girls concert at the Woodland Park Zoo in Seattle. After settling into a decent viewing spot on the lawn of this festival-seating venue, I make my way through the throng toward the line of portable rest rooms. It's a sold out show and it is nearly time for the performance to begin, so as expected I find maybe 50 people already in the queue. However, there are approximately 7 units with a larger wheelchair accessible one on the end closest to me, so turnover is quick and presently I find myself at the head of the line.

A woman with a cane makes her way slowly past everyone else and positions herself behind me. She is accompanied by another woman.

"Hello," she greets. We'll just stand here, right behind you."

"I assume you're waiting for the one on the end?" I reply, trying to tactfully imply the wheelchair accessible unit.

"Yes, but you take it if it opens first," she says amiably.

I don't quite catch on and I give her a confused look.

"You do know that you can just pass all these people and go right to the head of the line?" she offers helpfully.

It dawns on me what she is talking about.

"But I'm not…" I start, without thinking. I catch myself, concerned that I'm being politically incorrect.

As I finish with the word "disabled," it is lost under her answer. "It's OK, honey. Took me nine years to be comfortable with that."

I mutter something about her having a cane, hoping I'm not being rude, but thinking to myself that if I qualified for a disabled parking pass then it would be more logical to assume I could go to the head of the line to use the restroom. I am genuinely puzzled as to why this woman would think that my different face should grant me this privilege.

I am saved further conversation by a stall opening up, which I am all too eager to occupy to make good my escape. It happens to *not* be the wheelchair accessible one. I am not angry because I understand that she is trying to be helpful, yet I resent being judged for my face alone. She can consider herself disabled if she wants to, but it is a label I've chosen not to wear.

For the next several months, I rebelliously avoid the disabled stalls in any restroom I happen to be using. While I don't mind using my appearance to my advantage in some situations, I have my limits. I consider myself fortunate to have full use of my arms and legs.

Chapter Thirty Five
Taking Flight

Despite acquiring a lucrative position with the federal government, I don't immediately quit Dairy Queen, perhaps out of a misplaced sense of loyalty. But once the manager learns that I don't really need the hours, I am fazed out of the schedule in favor of people who need to earn a living. I take the hint and take my leave.

Our small work group consists of three audio visual specialists, three still photographers and two support staff. We are primarily made up of ex-military and people who qualified via DVR.

As a full time employee, I am making more money than I have ever seen before. Medical benefits are good and there are several plans to choose from. My cat and I move out of my parent's house for the final time into a small rental closer to work.

The audio visual team has several routine functions. We duplicate video tapes, maintain a video library, download educational satellite programs, document events on video, and produce training and educational programs. The types of events documented include visitations by VIPs, dignitaries and politicians, also known as "grip and grin" events. We cover annual or special events, including retirement parties, Pearl Harbor Day commemorations and group trainings. Some of the more interesting work includes video documentation of underwater systems and weapons testing.

The Naval Undersea Warfare Center, as it comes to be called after several name changes, manages several underwater tracking ranges, including one shared with Canada off the coast of British Columbia. This is a favorite destination, as it usually involves being shuttled around by various aircraft and watercraft, from helicopters to Navy frigates.

On one particularly memorable assignment, our crew is tasked with taking footage of a test torpedo which will be launched from a naval vessel. One of us will shoot from a helicopter and another from a smaller boat well clear of the launch path. I score the helicopter, which is the sought-after position because face it; I get to feel like I'm shooting an action movie. The sky is clear and the wind is calm, ideal conditions for the "helo" to fly safely and for taking video. As I wait near the helo with my stack of equipment, the pilot removes the door nearest where I'll be sitting. This is necessary in order to get a clean shot with no obstructions and to accommodate the long lens needed to shoot from that sort of distance. I'm wearing a bright orange flight suit made of thick warm material. I am sweating in it now, but I'll be glad for it once we are airborne. It is also a floatation device, so if we end up in the drink it could save my life. The air is cold up there and the movement of the helo creates its own chilling wind. I've learned on previous trips that when it comes to blowing hair around, convertible automobiles with the top down have nothing on helicopters in flight with the doors off. I have my hair anchored in place as best I can with an army of bobby pins, lest it whips my face and eyes like wire.

When the pilot signals that he is ready to depart, I climb in and rest my cumbersome equipment on the seat next to me. The camera is a Betacam, which is the type the news people use. The regular lens has been replaced by a long lens designed for shooting from a great distance and I've made sure I have a freshly charged battery and a new tape. When I start shooting, this massive assembly will sit on my shoulder held in place only by my arm. I don a headset so I'll be able to hear the pilot over the engine noise and the buffeting wind. After I am buckled in, the pilot wraps duct tape around the metal seat belt clasp. The strap remains adjustable, but we are increasing the odds that I will remain in the helicopter for the entire ride.

The rotors spin up to speed, and we lift off. The pilot finds our position and we wait for the launch. And wait. And wait some more. Helicopters are designed to hover, but it takes constant adjustments by the pilot to keep us in one place. We are pushed around and rocked by the wind. The wind may have seemed calm on ground level, but the gusts increase with elevation. As expected, I am glad for the warmth and protection of the survival suit. When word comes through my headset that launch is imminent, I hoist the camera with its extended lens to my shoulder, putting the camera's nylon strap around my body as a safety line in the event that it should somehow slip from my grip. The pilot takes us as close as he's allowed to be. I loosen my seatbelt strap, which allows me to maneuver to the edge of the seat and hang partially out the open doorway. The camera is heavy enough on its own, but with the addition of the supersized lens the assembly seems to weigh as much as I do. The weighty lens wants to tip the camera forward and it's all I can do to keep myself and the camera in position. Despite my best efforts to hold my hair at bay, stray strands break free and flog my face, stinging my eyes. My exposed hands are frozen, but I need bare fingers to activate the camera's controls. My fingers know the way around these controls even if their sense of touch is numbed.

I am constantly compensating for the continuous movement of the helo and the trembling of my limited strength, though the heaviness of the camera actually helps to keep it steady. But despite the specialized lens, zooming in on far away objects from a moving object makes for a shaky picture, so I am forced to keep the shot somewhat wide. When the torpedo finally launches after what feels like an eternity of balancing that monolith on my shoulder, I manage to keep it in frame, which is a noteworthy accomplishment. I wish the shot were closer in and of better quality, but I feel I did the best I could under the given conditions.

On the way back, we spy a pod of killer whales.

"Can you take us any closer?" I implore hopefully, shouting into my headset's microphone. *What a nice opportunity to get some rare footage.*

"I'm only allowed to get so close," the pilot responds. "Regulations."

But the creatures seem so far away through the lens.

The helo sweeps in and I capture some footage as these mammoth creatures glide gracefully through the water. A few of them rise up in full vertical breech and I am lucky to capture those images as well. It is only when I take my eye away from the viewfinder that I discover how close we actually are to those whales! They appear further away through the camera and I realize the pilot has definitely fudged the rules for me. I thank him profusely, hoping he won't get into trouble for doing so. The quality of the footage is nothing you would see on National Geographic, but I am elated to have had the opportunity to try.

When it comes to the production of educational and training programs, I am a one man show. I write the scripts with the help of the project manager, shoot the footage and edit the program together. I find voice talent from within the Center staff and direct them as well. Most of the projects are dry and straightforward, but they accomplish their goals and make the clients happy.

I have some decent equipment to work with. My only option is linear editing, so once a shot is laid onto the master tape,

I'm pretty much stuck with it. If I want to change the timing of any of the shots, I have to re-edit all the material that comes after. If I want to replace a shot with a different piece of footage, I have to replace it with a segment exactly the same length and redo any transitional effects.

At the end of each fiscal year, some of the codes (departments and sub-departments) need to spend money quickly. If they fail to spend all the money they are given, they get less the following year, so we are often the benefactors as codes shed their extra dollars. When we are gifted a newer fancier edit controller, a training seminar is included in the price and I am sent to the American Film Institute in Los Angeles to learn how to use it. Since I've already earned a college degree, I've given up my dream of going to school here on a full time basis, but am thrilled to be able to visit and take a training course on the campus. I achieve my goal of attending AFI after all, albeit not in the educational capacity I'd originally hoped.

While in Los Angeles, I take the opportunity to reconnect with Lena, who is too busy for me. She has her profession to pursue, but it is nice to see her again if only briefly and to thank her once more for her kindness.

Chapter Thirty Six
Continuing Education

At my Federal job, I have a friend and ally named Ben who is not only an acquaintance of my father, but also happens to be the department head for one of the largest and richest codes. Since I do a lot of projects for his programs, his department pays for me to attend a continuing education course on video production at the University of Washington.

Ben also happens to be on the board of directors for a small community theater which produces exclusively musicals. Since I am single with no social life and with lots of extra time on my hands, Ben offers me a creative outlet that will allow me to exercise abilities I already possess as well as expand my knowledge and experience.

It is late summer, 1990. I drive into the dilapidated remains of downtown Bremerton to keep an appointment with Ben and begin a long term commitment to community theater.

This metropolitan area was once the center of shopping for Kitsap County, but when the new supermall opened in Silverdale in 1985, the department stores vacated these buildings, leaving gaping empty vandalized holes off semi-deserted streets. After finding a place close by to park, I enter the old Sears building, its large display windows flanking the entrance. The main floor is gutted, leaving an ample open area to be divided between performance space and audience. I find Ben working on wiring and he greets me as I enter.

"You made it," he says.

He finishes up what he is doing and gives me a quick tour,

not that there is much to see. He then leads me over to introduce me to Christopher, theater founder and director of the current production, *Carousel*.

"Dawn is the one I told you about who is interested in helping with lights," Ben tells him.

"As you can see by this mess, we can use all the help we can get!" Chris responds.

Christopher is middle-aged, bald, and takes the old theatrical saying "the director is god" literally. But I soon discover he has the talent to back up the ego. He is demanding, and I eventually learn to filter out his tirades, especially since they are often aimed at actors who haven't learned their lines or support staff who haven't performed to expectations and are therefore usually well-deserved. I see him reduce people to tears, which is uncomfortable to watch but better than being at the receiving end. Yet Christopher is respected and many who work with him are fiercely loyal and return show after show. I come to understand that he is a perfectionist and expects those around him to deliver in kind. He has a gift for getting what he needs in both the physical sense such as set pieces and props as well as in performance from his actors, costumers, set builders and crew. For these reasons, his productions are quite the spectacle, despite limited resources.

Like most community theaters, this one is under-funded and always in need of volunteers. And, just like at the university, most people who get involved want to perform on stage, so having someone who is dedicated wholly to technical support is more than welcome.

I spend many hours with Ben and Christopher getting the technical aspects of the show ready. I become Ben's primary assistant for many of the tasks that require his engineering expertise. We hang metal piping from the ceiling in order to have a place to clamp lights, as well as find a way to run cables and wiring in such a way as to not interfere with the performance and to not be under the feet of the audience.

Chris views me as a mixed blessing. On one hand, I can help with tasks he would otherwise have to do himself. However, teaching a newcomer such as me how to do these things initially costs him more time than he saves. It turns out to be a worthwhile investment as I become one of his loyal subjects and a mainstay in the company for several years.

Between Chris and Ben, I learn how to read a written light plot. I am shown how to hang the lights, lock them into place, and how to focus the beam to create even lighting in the desired areas. I slide colored gels in front of each light which help affect the mood of each scene. They teach me that lights are connected on circuits, which allow certain groups of lights to come on at the same time using a single fader on the light board, so which lights plug into which circuit has to be carefully planned out.

What excites me the most is that Chris teaches me what my paid educators would not: how to be a light board operator. I will run lights for every performance of *Carousel*, which I will do from the back of the house.

"Don't slam the dimmer up so fast!" he yells from front-of-house. "Feather it gently!"

Chris eventually takes my education even further and teaches me light design. What had been so incomprehensible in a university classroom becomes much easier to grasp in this real-world setting. I become his apprentice, learning by doing.

Since my presence is required at most rehearsals, I spend a lot of time around the cast, crew and other creative forces in the production. Since there is virtually no technical staff, Chris mandates that the cast pitch in at work parties.

It is in this cast that I meet someone in whom I take a romantic interest. He catches my eye, even if I fail to catch his.

Chapter Thirty Seven
Emotional Spin-Dry

My romantic history isn't anything to brag about.

I lose my virginity to a man significantly older and already in a committed relationship. Our affair begins innocently enough. We are in the same environment, which allows us to get acquainted and develop a rapport.

His name is Raymond and I am waiting for him like I do most days, on the street corner along the path he regularly takes. There are people about, and my eyes search through them in the direction he'll be appearing. I glance at my watch. Could be any time. I shift from one foot to the other impatiently. I feel so obvious, but I am captivated by him, craving his conversation and his company. He occupies my thoughts to the point of obsession. I check my watch again. Only a few minutes have passed, but I start to worry. What if he stayed home sick today?

Ah, there he is! I spot him in the distance and relief washes over me. Even as I try to act casual, my heart pounds in anticipation.

"Well hello there," he greets me with a smile. We walk together as we do nearly every day. He is not a handsome man, but the more time I spend with him the less it matters. It is his mind that captivates me. My attraction to Mick at the university was based primarily on looks, and that certainly didn't get me anywhere. I ponder the hypocrisy, that I should value appearance while I expect others to overlook mine.

Several weeks ago I met Ray's wife at a party they were hosting. Though I am attracted to her husband, I met her with a clear conscience as there was nothing going on between me and Ray aside from being friends. I got along with her just fine. In fact, meeting her made me feel even closer to him.

He is a gentleman toward me and though he seems to enjoy my company, I have no idea if my attraction to him is reciprocated. It is easy for me to assume it is all one-sided, since it always has been before. The very notion that someone could be attracted to me is completely foreign. I've had plenty of male friends and I've been attracted to a number of them, but the attraction has never been reciprocated either because they are gay, had girlfriends, or because they were just not interested in me romantically.

I feel elation as I walk with Ray. Being with him makes me less lonely and I look forward to our time together. I mostly listen, not always sure what to say. I often find our conversations intellectually challenging, yet I'm not as quick-minded as he is so sometimes I feel intimidated by what I perceive as his superior intellect. However, he makes me laugh and I am a sucker for a sense of humor. I interject when I feel I can add to the conversation. Sometimes we just walk in silence. But he touches my insecurity too. Am I smart enough to engage him or do I come across as a complete dufus? Does he find me even a fraction as interesting as I find him?

My heart begins to sink as we approach the place where we must part company. I subconsciously walk slower so as to not get there quite as quickly, but the moment inevitably arrives. I struggle for something to say that might keep him with me a few moments longer, but I can only stall for so long. I feel an ache as he departs. I watch him for a moment, then tear myself away from that spot to make my own way home.

Not many days later, I reach a decision. I'm going put the friendship we have forged at risk. I meet up with him as usual, but today my heart is in my throat for the entire walk, and it isn't until the end that I muster up my courage. I make sure that no one else is in earshot.

My brain is barely able to organize the words and my tongue trips as I stammer out the question.

"Are you interested in a physical relationship?"

This is not an intellectual decision. This is an emotional one. I have chosen to put the fact that he is married aside. This is not about her. This is about *me* and about Ray.

He lights up in response. "Really?" he says boyishly. *I thought you'd never ask.*

What about her?

It is better that she not know.

(Well, duh.)

It is his betrayal, not mine. If he is willing to take this step despite her, that is his choice. This is how I justify it. My conscience tells me it is wrong, but my own desperate need and passion are stronger than my ethics. My emotions are in charge. If he had said no the rejection would have been debilitating, but I would have tried to respect his answer and not push. It would have taken time, but I'd have gotten over it.

But he doesn't say no. *He wants me.* I am filled with excitement and anticipation. I want to experience the body that goes with that brilliant mind that I have become so infatuated with. *Finally, a chance at a physical relationship!*

Because he has become interested in me as a person, he is able to see past the face to the mind and body, the latter of which he is now free to openly admire, at least when we are alone.

He is careful not to rush things. He expresses his desire, but he never pushes me. When we kiss and caress in secret hidden places prior to our first sexual encounter, I see his facial expression change and feel his erection which both baffles and thrills me. *Someone desires me!*

My first time is on the front seat of his car. There is nothing magical about it. Instead, it is painful and awkward, despite how gentle he tries to be. Rather than reveling in ecstasy, I am impatient for it to be over.

Then it's done, by someone I care for and who cares about me. Not love, but not out of sympathy either. Genuine desire that I could not find amongst my peers.

"It gets better," he promises.

After years of deprivation, I can't seem to get enough.

"You are so young and tender," he proclaims in passion. And I am all the more happy to give myself to him.

Yet the more involved we are, the needier and more attached I become. My inexperience with these moods and sensations becomes a burden for us both. I simply do not know how to handle these new feelings in my body and in my head. It's as if someone has thrown me in the dryer and set me on spin dry, jumbling all these emotions and tossing me painfully in different directions.

Our time is limited due to him being married, and I consequently become clingy. Though we do a few things together, we cannot show our affection for each other publicly. No dates, no romance. Yet I crave these things.

The aching in my heart when we part company increases, and my efforts to deliberately delay his departure intensify. My loneliness is so great sometimes I cry. I know he finds this bothersome and at times worrisome, wondering what fatal attraction he's gotten himself into. He accuses me of having unrealistic expectations. I daydream about having a life with him, and though I voice it to him once or twice, he gently explains that he wants to maintain his marriage. It's the answer I expect, and in the recesses of my intellectual mind I know it would never work anyway. He is much older than I, and I have too much life ahead and too much ambition. I don't think our personalities would be compatible over the long haul either.

Despite this roller coaster of emotion which I can't rationalize my way out of, I manage to remain productive in other areas of my life. My projects and my work do not suffer.

I occasionally socialize with him and his wife, during which times I have to be guarded and to try to act dispassionate. Most likely she sees right through me but for her own reasons chooses not to make an issue of it. Maybe he has been able to convince her that my feelings are all one-sided.

We are successful in our discretion. If others suspect, they don't let on.

There isn't anyone I can tell for fear of gossip, but it is a difficult secret to keep. I want to share with the world that I have found someone, but I can't. Besides, he's not really *mine*. While I am not ashamed to be involved with a married man, I understand full well that this is not socially acceptable. I am determined not to be a home-wrecker, and promise myself that no matter what happens I will not be vindictive.

The age difference weighs on my mind as well. Another social stigma, but it helps to emphasize the impermanence.

Three years later, I excitedly announce to Ray that I've taken an interest in someone else. I consider Ray to be a friend with whom I can share my thoughts. His response is one of disappointment with a hint of anger.

"So I'm being cast aside because you're tired of me?"

His reaction surprises me. Our relationship has been winding down, the intensity waning. Or so I'd thought. I regard him in puzzled silence. Though I don't express it aloud, I can't deny that he is right. I suppose it is unreasonable to expect him to be happy for me, but I figured our gradual growing apart was mutual. *He has a wife, this has been a dead-end relationship for me, and he's jealous because I want to move on?*

Of course, it's not like I am progressing to anything nobler.

Chapter Thirty Eight
Another Woman's Man

Craig's office is plain. The walls are bare and white, the carpet is short and beige, and the furnishings consist of a sturdy work table, storage closet, another desk which sits unused and empty, plus a few extra chairs. His desk is basic, its most prominent contents being a computer and a phone. The office space is designed for workers on temporary assignment, so personal items are scant. I am sitting on the edge of the spare desk and Craig is pivoted in his chair, facing me, and we are engaged in a playful banter. I've been hired on as a short-term temporary at his place of employment. It's after-hours for me, but I often migrate there during the workday as well if things are slow. He's on a longer shift than I am, but I enjoy our visits enough to stay. I don't have much else going on in my life anyway.

I have realized that he has become foremost in my thoughts and I am drawn to his companionship. It's been a long time since I've experienced the giddiness of a new attraction.

We are the only ones in the building, and our playful banter has graduated to mild flirtation.

I become suddenly aware of a heaviness in the air that is unfamiliar to me. It tingles electrically and I reach for some way to identify it. Then it hits me.

Sexual tension!

I don't remember experiencing this with Ray. Most likely it was naïveté and ignorance, but I did not clue in to any reciprocation of my feelings. Up until the time I got up the courage to ask him point blank, I had no idea if he had any interest in me sexually. This time, I can see the change in Craig's expression when he regards me. Not necessarily lust, though there may be some of that. More like curiosity. Or longing. I am delighted by this; thrilled that I am able to recognize it, and that having someone be sexually attracted to me isn't just a one time occurrence. Even better, Craig is in his 30's, so only a decade separates us in age as opposed to the much wider spread previously. I feel better knowing I can attract someone younger if not quite my age.

Since I am so convinced our interest is mutual, I am able to more easily broach the subject with him.

"Under different circumstances, you and I could be more than friends," I suggest boldly.

He regards me with that familiar look.

"Yes, I suspect we could."

That out of the way, we are able to discuss our feelings more openly with one another. Unfortunately, there is the small matter of his wife and children, and I'm still involved with Ray. Initially at least, we are both reluctant to act on our attraction.

But the scintillating stirrings of a new relationship are a strong draw and eventually temptation gets the better of us. Craig and I arrange a time and place where we can be alone and undisturbed. My feeling regarding his marriage is that it is his choice to make, but because he has children my own twinge of guilt is stronger.

"Are you sure you want to do this?" I ask, looking into his eyes. It is an unfair question to ask a man with an erection, but I ask it with genuine sincerity.

I believe this to be his first extramarital affair. I cannot say what causes a good family man to stray, but I can say it has nothing to do with pity. Maybe there is a void in his life that needs to be filled, in which case if it wasn't me it would likely be someone else.

I'm fine with it being me. His interest and infatuation gives me confidence. I have two lovers now, proving that it is possible for men to become interested in me as a person, see past the face, and then desire me sexually.

Meanwhile, I knowingly traverse from one dead end to another. This ending is even more imminent, as I'll be moving before long, yet the knowledge that this is temporary is not what drives my actions. I am giving in to the emotional pull of the mutual attraction. After years of deprivation, I am reveling in the attention, and a part of me feels that I deserve this. Overall my emotions are more under control with Craig. I still feel deeply and passionately for him, but this time I am less needy and desperate. While not quite as casual as "friends with benefits," it's definitely less intense and I feel more in the driver's seat.

For a short while there is some overlap between Ray and Craig. I have a hard time feeling too guilty about this, considering both men are using me to cheat on their wives. But soon after Craig and I become more intimately involved, I lose interest in maintaining a sexual relationship with Ray. It's more a habit than anything I gain real pleasure from any more, and besides it makes me feel promiscuous and that's not the type of person I want to be, so I cease being sexually available to him.

Once again, circumstances dictate that Craig and I cannot have a proper courtship and that our communication is restricted. The closest we are allowed to a "date" is lunch as friends. Once again I am determined not to be a home wrecker and we are careful that his wife never gets wind of anything. We both know it cannot and will not last. Aside from his family, there is still a significant gap between us. While I find him interesting, sensitive and intelligent, he is not college-educated. It is not that I feel intellectually superior. Rather, we lack a significant common experience.

The inevitability of my departure offers us both a safety net. Not that his infidelity can ever be undone, but at least it will not be perpetuated. Not with me, anyway. This makes me feel a little less guilty, thinking that he can go back to his family when I leave. Perhaps my view is naive.

After I move, I expect that our relationship is done. I grieve our separation, feeling suddenly very lonely. I miss the intimacy, I miss the sex and I miss being desired.

The first time he calls me, I am truly surprised. Sure, I gave him my phone number, but didn't really expect to hear from him. I am uncertain what drives him and don't understand why he is reluctant to let it end, but I am flattered that he is still interested. I can justify visits as I have other friends and connections in town, so we share several intimate reunions. In retrospect, his act seems desperate. I come to realize that his need is greater than mine. I enjoy being wanted, since it hasn't happened to me before, but for me our relationship ceases to be fulfilling. I've lost the passion and our last time or two together I feel more like his diversion than his lover.

Did I love these men? Since I have no prior experience, I have no idea what it feels like to love or be in love. I experience deep, intense attachment, especially with Ray. Where are those lines between infatuation, need, desperation, lust and love? I believe that I loved Ray. I do not believe that he loved me, though I believe he cared for me as one might a close friend. I do not believe I was in love with Craig, and I was definitely more ready to move on than he was. I don't think he loved me either but his obsession with me, or at least with whatever I represented, was far longer lasting. He continued calling me periodically for several years.

It is important to note that in both of these relationships, we became friends *first*. In each case, we responded to a mutual attraction. This gives me confidence that despite the potential deterrence of my face, it is possible for men to be attracted to me. This also reinforces my conviction that more surgeries are not necessary. Men who find me interesting do so largely because they appreciate my intensity, energy, intelligence, thoughtfulness, straightforwardness and sense of humor. It helps that I am height-weight proportional and have a curvy figure. But then, the more time someone spends around me, the less they notice my appearance. My face simply becomes part of my identity.

I come to the conclusion that all it really takes is time for a man to get to know me, and then he'll find out how wonderful I am in so many other ways. I subscribe to the belief that I can and will be loved. I just need to find the right sort of man.

I ponder why so far it seems that only older men in committed relationships find me attractive. I suspect mature men are more quickly able to get past the asymmetry of my face and appreciate other physical and mental attributes. Maybe they consider me safe; since I'm not pretty their spouses or significant others are less likely to suspect them to be physically involved with me. Maybe they just want the sex they are deprived of at home, the thrill and danger of sneaking around, or maybe they are trying to tap into my youth and energy. Yet I never felt that either one of them were taking advantage of me. In both cases, I was the one that broached the subject of a more intimate relationship first.

On a more ominous level, sex becomes for me a sincere way of expressing affection. I allow the friendship to be taken to a different level because I am hungry for the intimacy.

But I'm tired of sneaking around. I really want someone of my own.

I can't seem to find any younger, single, available men willing to spend time getting to know me. Maybe men my age aren't mature enough to get past appearance. Maybe they consider me to be bad for their image; it's too important to them to have some babe draped on their arm. Maybe they haven't made enough mistakes with the pretty women yet to realize looks aren't everything. Or maybe it is a mere matter of exposure. A common theory states that if you want to meet the right sort of someone, you have to go out and do the things you enjoy. In these places, you meet people of like minds.

I started volunteering in community theater not to meet guys, but because I enjoy the work. This exposes me to a whole new group of like-minded people. So if I am approaching things the right way this time, how do things end up so terribly sideways?

Chapter Thirty Nine
Jigger

The cast member of *Carousel* who catches my eye is portraying Jigger. How fitting it should be the role of the antagonist.

Max is average height with thinning dark hair and a mustache but rather gaunt features. He is thin, except for the makings of middle-aged spread. He doesn't show any interest in me.

Asking around, I find out that he is living in Christopher's basement, so I ask Chris about him.

"Hon, he's in the middle of a divorce. You don't want to get mixed up with someone on the rebound. Besides, he's a druggie."

"Isn't he in rehab?" I naively ask, thinking that makes everything better.

"Well, yeah. An out patient program. Part of his effort toward reconciling his marriage."

"You think that will happen? Reconciliation?"

"I don't know. Doubt it. His wife already has a new boyfriend."

It doesn't occur to me to ask whether the rehab program is actually working for him.

I hang out with him anyway, as opportunity allows. He is cordial enough towards me, but still shows no interest.

My attraction to him defies logic. He isn't bad looking, but nor is he especially charismatic. We hardly talk, and therefore don't even form anything that could be considered a friendship. What little I do know indicates we don't have much in common. But I push aside these things because I am lonely to the point of desperation, and since reconciliation with his soon-to-be ex-wife unlikely, he is more or less available.

I consider him a project. I view him as a recovering drug addict seeking to make a positive change in his life and I naively believe that I can make a difference. Perhaps if he has someone around who is a good example it will inspire him to stay clean. How am I to know he's in the bathroom during performances snorting cocaine? Chris would have his hide if he knew. Or maybe he does know but what can he do? Max shows up for rehearsals and performances, and there are no understudies in community theater.

My entire social circle revolves around this show. Most of the cast members are great and I make a few friends, but I crave something more intimate. So after a Saturday night performance near the end of the show's run, I put one final effort into getting Max's attention.

I arrive at Christopher's door. It's late, but I can tell he is still up by the lights on in his house. The basement is only accessible from inside the house, so I knock. Christopher answers the door and greets me.

"Is Max around?" I ask.

"Yeah, he's downstairs. I think he's in bed already."

"Can I go down there?"

"Sure, I don't care."

"Thanks."

I proceed down the stairs a bit nervously. I already know what I intend to do. The basement is small. There is barely room for the queen sized bed, dresser, and a large television. A small bathroom is off to one side of the stairs. Clothes and belongings are strewn about. Max, as predicted, is already in bed. His shoulders are bare.

"Max?"

"Huh."

"You awake?"

Another grunt.

Shaking, I completely strip down. I've never offered myself in this way before. I feel cheap, but stubbornly continue. It is easy to stand back and say *if he isn't attracted to you as a person, why would you want him to have you in this way?* Because I believe that if he can get past my face, I have an attractive body. If I can get his attention any way possible, maybe the rest will follow.

Leaving my clothing in a pile behind me, I glide over to the bed and roll him over.

His eyes widen. He's awake now, and I have his attention.

"Whoa," he mutters.

I peel back the covers to discover he sleeps commando, so I straddle him. However, though his eyes are feasting on me and his hands are active, he remains limp in one vital area. Despite my best efforts, and his, nothing happens.

"It's the cocaine," he confesses.

"What?" I reply. "I thought you weren't doing that anymore."

"It was just a little bit. It wasn't mine. David brought some. I needed it to get through the show."

"Aren't you in rehab?"

"I am. I'm not going to do drugs anymore. It was just this one last time."

I want to believe him so I let it go. Yet again I stubbornly shut up the warning voices in my head that are trying to tell me *this is a bad idea.*

By then, it is around 2 AM. I climb back into my clothes, not sure whether to feel frustrated or smug. He noticed me, but I have no idea if it will have any lasting effect. I climb up the stairs in hopes of not waking Christopher and let myself out.

Chapter Forty
Walking Through a Storm

Max still occupies my thoughts, but nothing seems to have come of my effort. With no foundation of friendship to bond us, I resolve to give up and let this one go. *Carousel* closes and several weeks pass.

He comes knocking on my door one afternoon, totally unexpected and unannounced.

"Hi," he says. "Look, Chris needs me to move out of his basement and I remember you had some interest in me. I wondered if I could stay here for a few days."

Lonely and happy to see him, I am flattered that he would seek my help. I acquiesce with almost no hesitation, once again slamming silent the warning voices in my head.

Things go smoothly enough and I am glad for the company. I enjoy having someone to take care of. After a few days, he asks if he can stay longer. We come to an agreement on rent and I help him move his stuff in.

His bed takes over my small dining room with his dresser alongside, and his large television adorns my living room since it is more substantial than the one I have. He works in Seattle as a driver doing food delivery, so he earns a pretty decent wage, but he never seems to have any money. In fact, he takes an advance on his next paycheck.

"How are you ever going to get ahead if you keeping drawing off your next paycheck?" I ask him incredulously after he informs me of this.

"I need the money now," he insists. "There are debts that can't wait."

"What about your bills? Can they wait?"

"They'll have to."

"What the heck are you spending your money on?"

"Look, I owe someone money and it has to be paid or else I'll be in big trouble."

I don't know how to address this issue.

I remain financially independent of him, maintaining my own bank account. I am still working at the Naval Center at this time, so my finances are stable. My salary is more than ample to cover living expenses. The household bills are under my name and I make sure everything gets paid. I pay the rent and buy the groceries. Since I've been raised to be fiscally responsible, I don't understand his constant debt, even when I learn that he is still spending money on drugs.

Creditors start calling for him. Overdue notices on his bills arrive in the mailbox. His bank account is constantly overdrawn and the overdraft fees are starting to pile up. He consistently neglects to pay the rent he owes me and I allow him to get away with it. About the only contribution he makes to the household are food items that he brings home from work. When I question him about these, he says they are near expiration and the company will throw them out anyway. I don't know if this is true or not.

"Let me take over your finances," I suggest. "Give me your paycheck and I'll make sure all your bills are paid."

He agrees. I start by loaning him the money to catch him completely up on his debts so he'll start fresh.

Obviously I don't yet understand the power of addiction.

"You're enabling him," says Christopher, who has remained a mutual friend.

"I need to give him another chance," I respond, still thinking I can be the hero and save Max from himself.

"Codependency will do that to you," Chris replies.

But these are my choices to make and my lessons to learn. Chris knows this and all he can do is stand back and watch as I bury my head in the sand.

The first month, Max does give me part of his paycheck. Not enough to cover all his bills, but I stretch it as far as I can, supplementing the rest with my own money. This includes child support for his two young daughters.

One day I come home from work, walk through the door, and have the sudden sense that something is missing. The living room looks slightly larger, and I quickly realize it's because his large screen television is absent.

"Max, where is your TV?"

"I hocked it," he responds matter-of-factly. "Don't worry, I'll get it back next paycheck."

"Are you kidding me? Like you don't have enough debt?" I bail it out for him, this first time. It is not long before it disappears again, eventually for good.

For Max, the marijuana, alcohol, crystal meth and cocaine are higher priorities than his own obligations and debt. When he is either laid off or fired from his job, I'm not sure which, he resorts to collecting unemployment to pay for his drugs. The dealers always get paid first. I can only watch his self-destruction with frustrated anger and sadness.

When he is home, he blares Christian music from the stereo, which has little appeal to me. He has talent on the saxophone and I enjoy when he plays, but more and more often the instrument is in hock.

I am not a victim, except of my own tolerance, loneliness and fear. I have allowed myself to become deeply attached to him, or if not him at least to having someone to take care of. But he has little or no regard for my feelings.

Sex seems to be the only way I can get the attention and contact I crave. Not that he is a great lover, but he is available and usually willing, when he is not inhibited by the drugs. He makes no effort to satisfy my needs. Desperate for his attention, I tell him to come to my bed whenever he wants.

One night, he wakes me out of a sound sleep, slithering into my bed and groping at me and rubbing on me. I glance at my clock and see that it is 2 AM, and I have to go to work the next morning. I grumpily point this out to him.

"You said any time," he defends.

But instead of being flattered by his attention, I am annoyed.

"Well, I take that back," I whine tiredly. "So get it over with and leave so I can go back to sleep."

"I like the darkness," he proclaims. "This way I don't have to see your face."

I am stunned that he would tell me this while lying on top of me.

"Well, that's not a very nice thing to say," is about all I can manage in response.

Then there are nights he doesn't come home at all, the meal I've prepared uneaten. I lay awake, hurt and angry that he has no regard for my feelings or appreciation for what I do for him. Yet I am also worried, knowing that he's out destroying himself with drugs. I even call the Crisis Hotline, but get no useful advice.

One afternoon, he exits the house towards his car. I know he's on a drug run, and a compulsion to stop him overwhelms me. I race out of the house after him.

"Max, don't go," I plead.

He ignores me, getting in the car and starting the engine. Without thinking, I jump onto the hood of the car. He looks at me as if I've lost my mind because I probably have, followed by a look of angry determination. He throws the car into reverse and starts backing up, forcing me to grab onto the rim where the hood meets the windshield. There isn't much to hold onto here. He picks up speed and I hold on tenaciously, now afraid to let go. He backs out of the driveway and onto the street, but thankfully aims the car toward what he knows to be a dead end rather than out onto the main road where there will be traffic. I find the ride oddly thrilling. It is scary but not terrifying, and though I do wish I had a better grip, I don't get the impression he's deliberately trying to throw me off. Rather, he wants to shake me up, literally and figuratively. He roars down the dead end road, does a three-point turn with me still firmly attached, and speeds back to the driveway, turning sharply in. From my perch I have no gage of speed. It's a good clip but probably not enough to do serious damage if I did roll off. I do get tossed around on the hood as he makes the turns but I manage to maintain my grip. He comes to a stop in front of the house again and I let go. I roll off the side onto my feet, shaking from adrenalin and over-extended effort.

"You are crazy!" he proclaims, but as soon as I am clear he stomps the gas and roars backwards again, leaving me standing there helplessly watching him go. I sob from frustration and failure, angry at myself for my own behavior and angry at him for leaving. It is not the only time I pull this stunt, but each time it gets progressively more dangerous. I finally resolve that it is ineffective, as are any efforts I make to curb his behavior. But I am still too attached or too afraid of my own loneliness to make any changes.

One day as I peruse my checkbook I notice that he has forged a check for $100, which he has cashed. Though I confront him, I let it go. Another time, he obtains my bank machine card and my pin and makes a withdrawal. I have to give him credit that it is a modest amount, not even equaling the daily withdrawal limit. I change my pin and become more guarded of my purse. Somehow he draws that line himself as neither type of incident is repeated.

When I share some of my written work with him, he belittles it. Nothing I do can please him; putting me and my work down is a form of control. He teases my dog and my cats. One time he chases one of the cats under the bed. I lose it then, screaming at him to stop and beating him with my fists like a mother protecting her child, months of pent-up frustration unleashed on him. He does not fight back, but he never chases my cats again, at least while I am home.

These are but a few examples of how intensely the emotions he invokes in me manifest. In another incident, I become frustrated and angry with him over some discussion we have, probably about drugs, money or the fact that he is taking advantage of me. I turn to exit the house. It's a warm day, and the wooden front door is open. The outer door is screen on the top and glass on the bottom, and it is closed. Focused internally on my anger, I reach for the metal handle to open the door, apparently with some velocity…and miss.

I am startled out of my ire by the sound of breaking glass. I look down to see my open fist, poised as it had been to grab the door handle, suspended on the other side of the door, my wrist even with where the glass had been. Broken glass is scattered at my feet. I hadn't felt anything. No impact, and certainly no resistance. It takes a moment for the reality of what I've just done to sink in. I've never broken boards in Karate, or anything else for that matter, but this experience gives me an acute awareness of how that's done. Max comes up behind me.

"I can't believe you just did that," he says. *Is that awe I hear in his voice?*

I bring my hand back through the hole. Blood forms where the glass has cut me, and I see it before I feel anything. Max cautiously helps me clean and bandage my hand. My dark mood has shattered along with the glass and I find myself grateful for his ministrations. It is one of the few times I ever feel a gentle touch from him. But such moments never last.

There is a childishness to him, and I have trouble interacting with him as a mature adult. He mocks my speech, turning the "s" to an "sh."

"Sho, Dawn, whatsh for dinner?"

"That's not funny," I respond, no humor in my voice.

"I only shpeak like thish it becuashe I nubsh you," he continues. "Nubs" is his way of saying that he has affection for me that is not love. In this context, it is a made-up word.

"Just stop. I don't like it when you talk like that. It hurts my feelings."

"It hurtsh your feelingsh?"

Another way to belittle and control me. I begin to comprehend that he is verbally abusing me.

He never pretends to love me. In fact, he makes a point of making sure I know he doesn't. He never kisses me. We never go out to eat. He tells me about other women he is interested in and has supposedly slept with. I never know what to believe since lying comes so easily to him. He admires my energy, once saying that he needs cocaine to keep up with me. I take it as a compliment. But then, he has reached a point in his addiction in which he needs drugs to do pretty much anything.

Though I have opportunities, I never try any of the drugs except for a joint now and then, only to discover I have no affinity for it. I sit for long periods in the car outside his dealer's house waiting impatiently for him to emerge and hoping that the cops don't pick that moment to do a much-deserved raid.

There is one incident in which I am cleaning the couch cushions and find a small packet about the size of my fingernail. It's too deliberate to be a random piece of trash so I take a closer look and realize it is part of the page from a pornography magazine folded into a pouch. Not having any idea what it is, I start to unfold it.

"Max, what is this?"

He looks over, as I continue unravel it, seeing a hint of white powder, and the next thing I know he comes flying across the room at me.

"Give it here!" he demands.

I reflexively twist away from him, but he knocks into me hard and makes a grab for the folded paper, ripping it from my grasp. It is gone up his nose even as its identity becomes clear to me: a hit of cocaine. I am surprised by the violence of his reaction, bruised by the impact, and disgusted at his desperation to take it from me.

I see through everything and am aware of the wrongness of it all, but still choose to do nothing about it.

Chapter Forty One
Wake Up Call

I am not happy with what I've become. Chris, a recovering addict many years sober, has provided me with the buzz words, but the acceptance of the truth takes time. I am an enabler and codependent to a drug addict. I place his needs above my own, I am the one exerting all the effort into what is primarily a one-sided relationship, and I tolerate his abuse. Chris had warned me from the outset that I would not be able to change him, but I had refused to accept that.

"The only way he has any chance to pull himself up is if he hits rock bottom, Hon, and he won't do that with you taking care of him."

I am attached to his presence and get some small satisfaction out of having someone to take care of even while I am being emotionally crushed. My family doesn't like Max very much and can tell he's not making me happy. My co-workers also know something isn't right, but since I won't talk about it everyone who actually does care about me is powerless to help.

While his mental abuse is becoming clearer to me, so far he has not physically assaulted me. But during a shouting match one night, he puts a dinner plate through the flimsy wall panel of the rental house. For the first time I am worried about my safety, so I call 911.

"My roommate is getting violent and throwing things," I whisper into the phone.

"Has he harmed you?" the dispatcher asks.

"No."

"Are there any children in the house?"

"No, just me and him."

"Did you just call the police?" he yells from the next room.

I hang up suddenly regretting having called. I hadn't given my address yet.

"You did, didn't you? My ex used to do that too." *Is that concern in his voice?*

"I'll cancel it," I say, dialing the phone again.

"I just called, but everything's OK now. I don't need you."

"OK, ma'am, we'll take care of it," the voice assures me.

I learn two things that night. The first is you can't cancel a 911 call once it is made. A patrol car arrives at my door a short time later.

"Is everything all right here?" the officer at my door asks.

"He started throwing things."

I want him to leave. I don't even mind if they take him.

"Has he harmed you?"

"No, but he put a hole in my wall."

"Does he live here?"

"Yeah, I pay the rent and he pays nothing, but yeah, I guess he does."

"OK, ma'am, if he lives here and he hasn't hurt you there isn't anything we can do."

It doesn't make sense to me that they would just leave me alone with him; someone who scared me into calling the police. *He may not have hurt me yet but how do they know he won't?* Thankfully, he is significantly subdued by their visit. He tells me that his ex-wife had called the police on him once as well, which tells me that violent behavior is not new to him.

I feel that a line has been irrevocably crossed. His behavior towards me is escalating toward violence, and I need to get out of this relationship while I still can.

They won't do anything because he lives here. That is the second thing I learn that night. Shortly after this revelation, I ask him to move out. He leaves peacefully enough, and for that I am grateful. But for added security, I get my family involved. I hadn't previously told them anything about Max's behavior toward me, his money issues, or his addictions because I'd been concerned they would only criticize me for keeping him around and I knew that this was something I had to work out on my own. Even though they didn't like him, they didn't bother me about him either. But now, I tell my dad everything, partially to make sure that I will follow through on getting this loser out of my life and partially because I know my dad, who is a rather imposing man, will help if I need him to.

However, even after Max is no longer living in my house, I can't quite completely let go. He finds a girlfriend, and despite seeing him treat her the way he treated me, I still feel jealous, and I hate myself for it.

He calls me periodically, usually asking for money. I don't give him any. He used my affection and interest to his advantage when he first moved in with me, and played my emotions as often as he could, yet slowly but surely, I am building up a resistance. I am getting over the emotional attachment.

He is living on the other side of Puget Sound, but he wants to come over for a visit, so I pick him up at the ferry. My parent's house is on our way out of town.

"I need to stop by my parents' place for a minute," I say.

"No, I don't want you to."

"It's just for a minute. You don't even have to get out of the car."

I make the corner and drive up their street.

"I said NO! I don't want to go there!" He is yelling now.

I ignore him, at which point he smashes the palm of his

hand into my face. I hit the brakes and turn to him in shocked surprise. I am speechless. He has never raised a hand against me before this, I am now in physical pain, and he could easily have caused an accident.

"Turn the car around," he demands.

I placate him by turning the car around, but this is the final straw. It finally sinks in that continuing this relationship in any form is not only unhealthy for me mentally, but he is increasingly crossing the line to physical violence. He is a user, and I have allowed him to use me. But I am done. After that incident, I sever ties with him completely.

There is, however, collateral damage. The relationship with my landlord, which had originally been cordial and even social, is irreparably broken. My landlord tells me he doesn't want his children to witness the sorts of altercations that occurred while Max was living with me, such as my wild rides on the hood of his car. I am confused by this, since Max has already moved out so such episodes are over. It crosses my mind that if he and his family had been witnessing these episodes, why didn't they approach me and offer to help? After all, we'd been on very friendly and social terms before Max arrived. I'd been through a rough patch, but instead of being supportive, my landlord turns hostile toward me. He raises the rent to a ridiculous level and I make the choice to move.

While Max owes me a good sum of money which I will never see again, I did allow him to put me into debt. Though he leaves me physically intact, I carry a few emotional scars, many unpleasant memories, and the periodic contemplation of how I could ever have been so stupid. But I am free of him.

It only took a year for me to find the strength to get out. Shorter would have been better and not at all would have been great, but I remind myself that this all started because I literally threw myself at him. Not that I deserved what followed, but I set myself up for it and allowed it to happen.

The experience provided some important education. I now better understand the physical, emotional and financial effects of addiction, but more importantly there is victory in having the self-esteem and wherewithal to break free.

Ironically, in the midst of my codependency, his ex-wife actually thanked me for preventing the steady spiral downward that he so richly deserved. Apparently, by keeping him afloat during the divorce proceedings, I prevented her from becoming responsible for vast amounts of debt. I'm glad someone was able to benefit from my fiasco.

I also facilitated him being able to see his two young daughters, even though he would leave them in my care while he went on drug runs.

One positive connection that is made through my relationship with Max is that I meet and become friends with his sister. She has a small farm and shares an interest in horses. Max probably also thinks we should get along famously because she has a scar on her lip that twists it a little, but I hardly notice. At any rate, she has a horse and some land, and proposes that I take advantage of a maintenance lease on a horse she knows named Toby. I jump at the chance, excited that after all these years I HAVE A HORSE! It's the realization of a dream.

Toby is an older Quarter Horse whose activity is somewhat limited from his history as a rodeo horse. He has a bad shoulder from always being required to cut one direction for the cow work he was doing, so he cannot handle strenuous exercise. He is an amiable gentleman, safe to ride and easy to control, and I'm a novice rider and not a daredevil so he turns out to be a good match for me.

For the first time in my life, I have a horse I am responsible for. Yet the fact that he isn't really *mine* hangs over me. Max's sister handles all his basic care, and all I need to do is come out and ride. However, since he lives some distance away from me, I find it difficult to spend a significant amount of time with him. Also, because I don't actively care for him, I fail to learn anything about basic horse care, except of course that I am required to pay his expenses. The romantic notion of finally having a horse doesn't captivate me for very long. I like him, I support him, but I don't form any significant attachment to him.

Despite this, and despite not having my own place to keep him, I contact Toby's owner and offer to buy him. My offer is turned down, as Toby is not for sale. I am disappointed at first, but shortly conclude that this may be for the best. He's an older horse with a chronic injury, and as he ages further there will be more expenses and maintenance to keep him comfortable, not to mention the question of long-term soundness. The last thing I need is to take on and pay board for a horse that I might in due time no longer be able to ride. With my life in flux, it's too soon for me to take on that sort of responsibility. After some thought of her own, Toby's owner calls me and offers to sell him to me but I express that I am no longer interested. Thus ends my first brush with horse ownership.

Too high maintenance and not enough return on investment. If only I had been able to apply such cool reasoning to my relationship with Max.

It is at his sister's house that I see Max one last time. She invites me to a small party at her farm. Most of her brothers, including Max, are present. He has been drinking, which is no surprise to me. A bunch of us are standing in the barn, when suddenly he pins me against a wall and begins grinding on me suggestively. An irrational terror takes hold, and I break out in a cold sweat.

"Max, don't. Stop it."

He is too physically close for me to knee him in the groin. At first, his sister and the others present completely ignore us, which I find disturbing and a little scary. But nor do I ask for help. Despite the increasing feeling of helplessness, a part of me struggles to find a way out of this myself without having to ask for help, while the other part silently hopes for intervention. Finally his sister looks over at us.

"Max, leave her alone," she says disgustedly.

To my relief he moves away, but after that I decide to make sure I am never alone with him.

Chapter Forty Two
A Man of my Own

The majority of the time that Max lives with me, I know it's a dead-end relationship. He has made it abundantly clear to me that I am not his girlfriend, so in an effort to explore the possibility of something more fulfilling, I take out a personal ad in the Little Nickel classifieds. I look damn good on paper. College degree, steady job in video production with a comfortable income, writer, horse lover, black belt in karate, light designer for a community theater, and on top of all that I am height-weight proportional. I receive several calls from interested parties.

I have no desire to waste people's time, just as I don't appreciate having my time wasted, so I decide to be up front about my facial features over the phone. I know full well this will mean that some callers will choose not to meet me.

The firefighter wants a babe, and turns me down at the mere mention of a facial difference. For him, it's all about image. Fine. At least he is honest about it. While I know I'm better off without Mr. Superficial, it pains me that he doesn't even offer me a meeting. But how can I complain when I'm the one who set myself up for it?

Mr. Athletic Bicyclist decides to keep an open mind and agrees to meet me, so I invite him over. It is instantly apparent that he is *so* not my type. He is tall, stringy, and almost too animated, but I'm willing to stifle my first impression and give him a chance the same way he gave me one. We chat for a while on my front lawn, made a bit awkward by Max choosing to pass through, undoubtedly on his way to obtain more contraband.

So that's two strikes against me from the outset- my appearance and a male roommate that I undoubtedly do a lousy job of hiding my feelings for.

"So do you have any interest in getting together again?" I ask halfheartedly as he prepares to leave, already knowing the answer.

"No, I don't think so. Sorry."

My disappointment at yet another rejection is fleeting. My complete lack of interest in him is the inevitable third strike.

Sadly this is as yet the closest I have come to being on a date.

In March of 1992 I am working on the light design for my community theater's production of *Music Man*. It's been a few months since I ejected Max from my house, but he is not yet completely out of my life.

It is not unusual for theater companies in adjacent communities to borrow from each other. Commodities such as props, costumes, furnishings, lights, actors, technical personnel, and directors tend to be shared, as the theater crowd travels in the same circles. Christopher has moved on, so a director who normally directs at Bremerton Community Theater (BCT) has been lured over to direct *Music Man*. BCT only presents one musical per season, while our theater devotes an entire season to them.

I am the in-house light designer and technician, so the design of *Music Man* falls on me. The director, having never worked at this theater or with me before, asks me if it would be OK to consult with my counterpart at BCT, whose work and knowledge she trusts. I agree. While I am working one weekend doing some final adjustments on the position of the stage lights, she invites him to the theater to have a look at my design.

We have long since moved out of old store fronts to our own building in the center of a nearby town. Many hours were spent by Chris, Ben, me and others to convert the space from a church to a performance theater. The recent second stage of remodeling and rewiring has elevated the lighting booth at the back of the house so it is only accessible by a steel rung ladder, which I am able to ascend and descend with grace and ease. From the vantage point of the booth, I see the director enter with a stranger in tow.

"Dawn," she says up to me. "This is Ian Shaw."

I am polite enough to him, showing off my design and the general workings of the theater, but little impression is made on me except that I think Ian is a cool name. My design passes muster with a few adjustments and the encounter passes from my memory.

By August I am free of Max once and for all. In the meantime, a producer has recruited me to design lights for BCT's production of *Nunsense*, their one musical of the season. BCT has been around since the 1940's, and it is successful enough to be able to afford much more sophisticated equipment including a more "high tech" lighting arrangement than what I am used to. The theater boasts a fly system, and a hydraulic lift to help designers adjust lights on bars trapped in place by set pieces. It has a catwalk above the house where large long-range lights are hung, and an entire wall is devoted to the dimmer system. I am definitely out of my depth, so in order to work successfully at this more complex theater, I need the help of their technician. This would be the same Ian Shaw, who serves on their board of directors as technical advisor.

He remembers me. I, however, have no immediate recollection of him.

There is nothing like spending hours in a theater hanging, focusing and gelling lights to get to know someone. The cast and crew of a show get to be pretty intimate from long hours spent together, often just waiting around for their turn to do something. Sometimes there is more drama behind the scenes than in the performance itself, including a considerable amount of pairing off with varying degrees of longevity. Technical people, however, often need to work when we have free access to the stage, so we work outside of scheduled rehearsal times.

On a Sunday, about mid-morning, I pull in to the parking lot behind the theater, pleased to see Ian's silver Volkswagen Rabbit already parked. As expected, there are no other cars. We've deliberately scheduled this time so we'll have the stage to ourselves. Actors come in handy for the final stages when we need to focus the lights, putting them in their final positions, but until then they would just be in our way. As I approach the door and punch in the key code which will allow me access to the locked building, I suddenly realize that I am looking forward to spending time alone with Ian.

Wow, that snuck up on me. I muse.

He's so different from anyone I've taken an interest in before. For starters, he's only two years older than me. More importantly, he's single. Though not unattractive, he is not a chick-magnet either. This may partially be due to possessing nerd-like qualities, many of which I find amusing and endearing. He recites lines from the original radio version of *The Hitchhiker's Guide to the Galaxy* and from *Monty Python* on a regular basis. He's intelligent, but is able to communicate the technical aspects to me in a way I understand. I can tell that if I didn't have some intelligence of my own, things might not be going as swimmingly between us. But that's not the only thing that attracts him to me.

We have the hydraulic lift, similar to what you'd see fruit pickers using in an orchard, out on the stage. It's my turn to go up on the lift to make adjustments on the light bar. I have controls on the platform and raise myself up. I hear him make an indistinguishable noise.

"What was that?" I inquire, thinking I might have missed something he said.

"Hmmm? Oh, nothing. Just admiring the view."

"So you're saying this is my better side?" I am enjoying the compliment.

"No comment," he replies. "Let's just say I noticed the same thing watching you go up and down the ladder when I came to check the light design for *Music Man*."

"Yeah, weird, I'd forgotten about meeting you there until you mentioned it."

"Well I didn't forget."

I find it flattering that he would remember me for my figure, most notably my derriere, rather than my face.

Ian works as an electrical engineer at Puget Sound Naval Shipyard in Bremerton. He is in the nuclear division, which is where many young engineers start out. He's been designing lights for BCT and been their technical board member for several years. *Nunsense* becomes the first of several shows that Ian and I co-design.

While we are working on the show together, we are mostly focused on the work. We have meals together because we are working long hours and we both need to eat. I would not consider any of those outings to be "dates." However, once the show opens and our work is basically done, we both know that this is not the last we'll see of each other.

I ask him if he wants to go with me to the Western Washington State Fair, and when he accepts this becomes our first date. There are two things of note. Firstly, this is not only my first date with Ian, but at age 26 this is my first date ever. Secondly, I am the one doing the asking. He insists he would have gotten around to asking me out eventually, but I'm not inclined to wait.

I am not feeling the intensity I've experienced with previous relationships. There isn't any electricity or explosive fireworks. Rather, we ease into our feelings gradually and they feel very comfortable, like a pair of shoes that fits the first time you put them on rather than having to break them in. Instead of flames, we feel warm fuzzies. I start spending a lot of time at his place, where we spend hours just lying in bed together, feeling the warmth and smoothness of each others' skin. Neither of us seems to have anything better to do with our time. He has no one else to go home to or to hide me from, and I revel in being the sole object of his affection.

He has had only one girlfriend before me, and that was fleeting. He felt very awkward with her. He describes her as clingy, wanting to monopolize his time, and he felt suffocated. I'm relieved that I got through that clingy stage with my first lover so I have a better handle on my emotions. Or maybe I am clingy too but he doesn't mind because he likes me better.

Standing in his kitchen, after knowing me for maybe two months, Ian makes a comment about us being together in the future.

"You may not still like me then," I quip.

"I think I will," he says philosophically. "I think whatever happens, we can work it out."

I look up at him abruptly from across the room. *Is that a hint of desperation I hear in his voice?* He's lonely, too. He's 28, and I've actually had more in terms of relationships than he has.

I experience a fleeting moment of panic at the notion of a long term commitment, quickly replaced by elation that someone could consider *me* in that context. *We really don't know each other very well*, I muse. *After all, we haven't been together very long!*

"I wonder if this discussion is a bit premature?" I reply hesitantly, then quickly add "not that I disagree…"

In the back of my mind I realize he is probably right. Even at this early stage, we both recognize that this could be a long term fit.

Later that year, I go with him to his 10th high school reunion in Connecticut where he grew up. We stay with his parents who are still living in the house he and his sister grew up in. To my amusement and dismay, we are put in separate bedrooms. However, after his parents go to bed I sneak into his room and crawl into his tiny twin bed with him. It's a tight fit but warm and snuggly on a chilly November New England night.

Given the nature of the trip, I also meet many of his school friends, from both high school and college. At a pub one night, after consuming a bit of alcohol, I get a little carried away with the idea that I finally have someone I can go out in public with. I embarrass him with a little too much public displays of affection. While I feel bad that it made him uncomfortable, I have a hard time feeling too sorry for him.

In May of 1993, his parents move across the country to a condo in Bellevue, Washington. Ian's dad informs him that he's put a bunch of his stuff from the house into a 1984 Honda Civic wagon, parked it at the neighbor's, and says if he wants it to come get it. So we fly out there and drive the car home. We stay for a few days to visit some of his friends, but then head south as there will still be snow on the northern routes. We take our time, and our itinerary includes Gettysburg, the scenic Blue Ridge Parkway, the Kentucky Horse Park, and the Grand Canyon. An empty theater gave us a chance to discover each other, but hours trapped in a car together on a long road trip put personalities to the test. It becomes the first of many road trips we will take together.

We both enjoy the companionship, finding in each other the end of years of loneliness and the comfort of being with someone who cares.

Chapter Forty Three
Electric Circus

Even though we met in a theater, I never have any expectation that Ian will behave like Max. In fact, Ian provides a stability I have not experienced in any relationship before, and I welcome this change. He has a job that pays better than mine. He is reliable, trustworthy and fiscally responsible and all his bills get paid on time. The idea that he might steal from me never enters my mind. I feel confident by this time that I would recognize signs of drug use or addiction, and Ian sets off no alarms. In fact, he doesn't even have expensive hobbies.

Ian appreciates that I have my own income, own my home and am also fiscally responsible. He admires my creativity and ambition, and unlike Max, who criticized any project I attempted, Ian is very supportive and encouraging. So when a professional writing opportunity comes up, he is happy to help.

I've kept in touch with a classmate from the continuing education course on video production I took at the University of Washington. Her name is Jenny, and we had worked on the same production team during the course and had really hit it off. We had decided to keep in touch not only because we like each other but because Jenny is active in production and could be a good professional resource. In the spring of 1994, I learn that she is producing an educational play for a public utilities district on the properties of light, geared toward grade school children.

Jenny is the co-founder and original artistic director of the Seattle Children's Theater. She is a vibrant individual, despite numerous health issues. She and the PUD commissioner have cooked up the idea for the play, calling it *Electric Circus*. She and I discuss it and she asks if I'd like to take a crack at the script. I'd have to do so completely on spec, which means not getting paid for the material I present. They already have a writer in Olympia under contract, but for whatever reason Jenny wants to see what I can do. I jump at the chance, eager for the opportunity to collaborate.

Jenny provides me with a concept outline. In *Electric Circus*, a troop of clowns demonstrates and explains the properties of light through various circus acts. Scenes include demonstrations of shadows, reflection, refraction, speed of light, splitting light, ROY G BIV (acronym for the colors of the rainbow) and ultraviolet light. She provides me with ideas for each scene as well as research material in the form of books so I have a better comprehension of what I'm writing about. Ian assists with the physics and the technical terms, as well as being a sounding board for the stories and comedy.

I have tight deadlines, so I worry about whether or not I can write creatively under pressure. However, I'm an expert procrastinator, so it is not unusual for me to be furiously working at the last minute regardless of what project I'm undertaking. The deadlines force me to park myself and write no matter what. I do not own a computer, but Ian does, so this has the added benefit of having to spend more time at his house. I am relieved to discover that not only can I be creative under pressure, but I can genuinely enjoy the material I am generating.

I do not consider myself an "ideas" person, but give me an idea and I can create from it, expand on it, extend it, and run with it. In doing so, I am capable of flickers of brilliance. But I do better with affirmation. I am grateful for Ian's moral support as well as his input. Unlike what I experienced with Max, Ian's feedback is constructive rather than derogatory.

Jenny and the decision makers at PUD are impressed by the samples I present to them. Apparently I have more accurately captured the spirit of their vision and the job of playwright is turned over to me. I am thrilled! To have my work produced is the realization of a dream. I am sure that my frequent and easy rapport with Jenny helped immensely but my ability to translate their ideas and blend them with my own creativity and humor is what earned their favor.

Electric Circus goes into production the following summer, and modifications are made due to technical necessity, budget limitations, or at the director's discretion. I am relieved that when Ian and I attend a performance, I can still recognize most of it as my work, and delighted to hear lines I've written and scenes I've crafted acted out before me.

I can now call myself a produced playwright, and if I wasn't considered so before, I am officially a professional writer.

Chapter Forty Four
Lighting up the Stage

After dating for approximately two years, Ian and I move in together. His lease has just expired, and I own my modular home in Suquamish, so he moves into my place. I am thrilled that we finally share the same home. We'd been commuting between houses and doing sleepovers, spending most of our time outside of work in each other's company anyway, so living together really doesn't require a huge adjustments. In fact, it saves time running back and forth. However, we know staying in my little house is temporary. His commute to work has increased substantially, and mine is about to.

Around this time, a woman I know through the model horse world needs to find new homes for her two ponies, and she offers one of them to me. The pony's name is Dancer, and she becomes the first horse I actually own.

Dancer is small, but I can ride her, and she is trained to pull a cart so I acquire a harness and two-wheeled cart and learn to drive. She doesn't take up much room and I can keep her in my backyard in what used to be the garden patch.

Dancer makes me realize that I know nothing about the practical aspects of equine care and maintenance. A simple task like giving her oral de-worming paste is clumsy and awkward. There are expenses that come with owning a horse that many people fail to consider, such as dental work, hoof care and vaccinations. It makes so much difference being responsible for arranging these necessities myself rather than relying on someone else like I did with Toby, the horse I had leased. Veterinary expenses can be high, because unless you have a truck and trailer, the vet has to come to you and they charge extra for that. I also learn after I acquire her that she has a progressive disorder known as Cushings disease. The physical signs are obvious to the trained eye, but since I didn't know how to recognize it when I first agreed to take her, this becomes another part of my education. I learn how to control her diet and she is on medication for the rest of her life.

Our family now consists of Ian, me, two cats, one dog and a pony.

The following spring, I get tired of waiting. At a Chinese restaurant in Bremerton, we are sitting at a table finishing up our meal.

"So, do you want to get married?" I ask somewhat matter-of-factly.

"Sure," he replies.

No romance. No bended knee. No proposal in a fortune cookie. We walk next door to the Fred Meyer and pick out rings. When I break the news to my mother, she fails to exhibit the enthusiasm I'd anticipated the news would bring.

"I thought you'd be happy to hear the news," I express.

"I am happy for you, honey," she explains. "But we've been expecting this so it isn't really a surprise. I'm sorry if you expected more of a reaction, but after all, you've been dating for… how long?"

Two years. Unlike Max, my family took to Ian very easily and everyone likes him. Our compatibility seems obvious.

We set the date for September 23, 1995.

As if getting married isn't enough of a change in my life, in July one of my co-workers hands me a classified ad for a video editing job in Olympia using the same type of editing equipment I currently use. The job is with a company that holds a contract with the state of Washington for video production. I create a resume and mail it in. After several interviews and on-site visits, I am hired for the position. It's a huge cut in pay but it will give me learning opportunities and practical work experience more advanced than what my often-boring government job can offer. I am most looking forward to working with an actual production crew. I am hired with the understanding that I am getting married and will be gone for a month on my honeymoon.

In September, shortly before the wedding, we move out of my modular home into a rental so I can be closer to my new job. This move shortens Ian's commute as well. Even though the stresses pile on between a new job, moving, wedding plans and travel plans, our relationship doesn't waiver.

Ian and I marry at the community theater where we first met on the production of *Music Man*. The current show is one that neither of us is working on called *Company*. A matte painting of the Brooklyn Bridge becomes the backdrop to our ceremony.

I am not interested in spending a ton of money on a wedding, so we cut corners wherever we can. Not that we can't afford it; we just see no point in having an expensive wedding. Since we are to be married in a theater, I make up the invitations to resemble a theater program, listing the cast of characters with Ian and I in the starring rolls as bride and groom.

A high school friend of Ian's is his best man. My man of honor is Murray. There is no one else I'd rather have fill this role.

Everyone is seated in the theater, and Ian's dad pipes us in on the bagpipes. Murray and I are on stage with the reverend and Ian and his best man are on the floor about to come on stage. Suddenly a man in the military dress uniform of an officer comes bursting loudly through the side doors into the auditorium.

"Um, excuse me," he says boldly.

"Can I help you?" asks the reverend.

"I'm here for the audition," he announces.

"What audition? This is a wedding," the reverend replies.

"I'm here to audition for the part of the groom," the officer states.

"Sorry," Ian interjects. "That role is already taken." His voice is shaking from nerves. I notice that his brow is wet with sweat.

"Oh. Too bad. I really thought I'd be perfect for the part. Are there any parts remaining?"

"We don't have a chauffeur," I inform him.

"Guess I'll have to settle for another bit part," he says. "Sure, I can be your chauffeur. I'll just have a seat over here and await my entrance."

He takes a seat.

The theater people don't bat an eye. They can tell that this has all been pre-planned. My then-brother-in-law tells me later he was ready to get up and toss the guy out, so not everyone keyed in. "The officer" is a friend from work whom I'd often used for voice-over narration in my video productions. He is a Naval Commander so the uniform is real. He conveniently owns a Jaguar convertible, so I had recruited him to drive us to the reception.

I am excited and nervous, but not nearly as nervous as Ian. I'm surprised he didn't blow his line.

After the reverend makes formal introductions, Murray plays a song on the harp and reads a poem that he had written especially for us.

I have written our vows, in which I name myself as Ian's "random element." I really am. Ian is content to sit in a house with all the curtains closed reading or playing guitar. Except for his work with the theater and role playing games with friends, he doesn't get out much. I consider it my duty to get him out of the house and into the world and I do a pretty fair job of it.

The entire ceremony lasts approximately 10 minutes, though it feels eons longer. Ian's dad pipes us out. We climb into the Jaguar and are driven away.

The harp and the bagpipes join us at the reception, which is held at a lodge by a lake. It is a rather ordinary reception otherwise, except for our wedding cake topper. Instead of the traditional bride and groom, we have two blown glass bighorn rams, butting heads. It's a private joke between me and Ian. We've developed a ritual of bonking our heads together lightly, maintaining the contact in what is more a gesture of affection than adversity, much like a cat might ram your leg with its head if it wants your attention. But on our wedding cake the rams also symbolize our understanding that we won't always agree on everything; that we will "butt heads" occasionally. I feel it's a pretty realistic way to enter a long term commitment.

Chapter Forty Five
Down Under

Since we are already living together, that is one adjustment we don't have to make. But being married feels different, like we've sealed the deal. Our commitment binds us, but in a happy, positive and constructive way.

Any money we saved on the wedding is splurged on the honeymoon instead. I've arranged for us to travel to Australia for a month. It is travel the way I like it- no concrete plan outside of renting a car and arming ourselves with an extensive road map and a travel guide or two. A month may seem like a long time, but Australia is a big country.

We have a week to transition from wedding stars to world travelers. After all the life changes we've recently endured, I am excited to escape with my best friend who is now my husband to a whole new wondrous world, free of obligation except to each other.

Our first night in Australia, after a crash course in driving on the opposite side of the road, we book into a hotel on Bondi Beach. After dinner, we go for a walk on the adjacent shoreline. In warmer months, this beach would be packed with surfers and sunbathers, but this early in the spring it is mostly vacant. Like its California counterpart, this stretch is very urban, and the buildings and pavement encroach as close as they dare to the sand and surf. We stroll along in the darkness, floundering through the finely ground sand until we discover that staying closer to the water is easier footing for tired feet. I love the solitude, alone in this dark foreign place with my man beside me, and I am so glad to be here on this great new adventure. Chilled by the wind, we hold hands, slipping both mine and his into Ian's pocket. I am warmed by Ian's company and soothed by the sound of the waves crashing onto a rocky point nearby. That night we sleep hard, fatigued by the stresses of travel and jetlag.

A few days later, after a pleasant day at the Taronga Zoo, we are on the bus back to our hotel, having opted for the ease of public transport rather than the stresses of driving and parking. A woman seated nearby addresses us.

"Enjoying your trip so far?" she inquires with an unmistakably American accent.

"Yeah, we are," we affirm. She is with a man, presumably her husband. They don't look at all familiar to me.

"We sat near you on the plane," she offers.

"Oh, OK," Ian responds.

I resist the temptation to roll my eyes. We hadn't had any interaction on the plane so it's not like we'd actually met. Ian shares my propensity to forget names and faces but there is no reason for us to remember this couple. They simply recognize me and my unforgettable face. I doubt they would have remembered Ian had he been by himself.

Ian does not share my love of horses and riding, yet riding a horse in Australia ala *Man from Snowy River* is on my dream list, so I've arranged for a guided excursion. This is northeastern rainforest instead of southeastern mountains but it will have to do. Ian has agreed to come with me, which I chalk up to both wanting to please his new bride and to being a good sport. I am grateful to him for not making me go alone.

Since I boast riding experience, I am given a skittish leopard-spot appaloosa gelding named Aztec who shies at everything while I am on the ground, but once in the saddle he seems to be fine. Ian mounts a roan mare named Misty, who is lazy and easy despite only being under saddle for three months.

She is rather small, but could be brumby and has no trouble packing Ian's moderate weight. She is safe and slow, but tends to prefer nibbling on anything she can get her lips around. At one point during the ride, however, she takes Ian under some tree branches, knocking his glasses and hat off. I watch helplessly, both concerned for his safety and frustrated that he hasn't taken more control of the placid beast to prevent her from doing that. Thankfully she fails to knock him out of the saddle, which is a relief to all of us, especially Ian. Our guide graciously dismounts and recovers Ian's belongings.

Two other women ride along with us, so we are five total. We ride through pastures, up and down steep hillsides on small dirt paths through grassy meadows that form a channel between brush and dense forest, across streams, through woods, along a dirt road, more wooded trails, more pastures, and on and on through this spectacular lush landscape. Though we both enjoy the scenery, Ian is just as glad to have this over with.

Knowing that we don't have time to see the whole country, we head south through Alice Springs to begin the loop back toward Sydney. Interested in exploring Ayers Rock and the Devil's Marbles, I book ahead for two nights' "budget accommodation" at Ashley Creek which is close to these tourist destinations.

When we arrive, I get a valuable lesson on first impressions.

Ashley Creek is a working cattle station with about 2-3 thousand head running on over a million acres, and they offer lodging as a sideline. When we pull in, there are a dozen or so locals stumbling or sitting about, peeing in the parking area, and climbing in and out of beater cars. These people appear a sorry lot. They are dirty, smelly and most of them are drunk. However, even so, these aboriginals seem less threatening than the aggressive panhandlers and barefoot bums of Alice Springs. Several even politely say "hello." But their presence makes me slightly uncomfortable and I begin to question the wisdom of staying here. I take in the rest of our surroundings.

The place itself isn't dingy. The grounds are well kept and the resident dogs are fat and lazy. This brightens me up a bit. At least the place is not neglected, and they obviously care for their animals. We check in and are taken to our room.

Our budget accommodation turns out to be a lumpy squishy double bed crammed into a shoebox with a dilapidated air conditioner which actually works despite appearances. At least it has a window. The room is part of a row of what looks like a trailer or single wide mobile home style units. They could be film-set dressing rooms, but Ian says they are military berthing. The bathrooms are in a separate building.

"At least we'll both fit on the bed," I note, trying to make light of my disappointment. In Tennant Creek days earlier we'd spent the night in twin beds, which just didn't seem right to me on my honeymoon. I felt like we'd been playing out a scene from *I Love Lucy*. Before that, we'd spent a night where we had to share a single twin bed, which harkened back to the visit we made to his parents when I'd snuck into his room. But then, snuggling up in a small bed isn't such a bad thing to have to do on one's honeymoon I suppose.

While the room by all appearances is fairly clean, the restrooms are disgusting. The shower has soap scum layers on its soap scum layers and I have to clean the toilet seat before I'll use it. I don't consider myself to be fastidious at all, but this pushes even my tolerance level. Even for the modest sum per night I expected better. I suggest upgrading to a more expensive room, but Ian is content with what we have. I don't argue with him since I'm not convinced that paying more would make a considerable difference, and it's not like we plan to spend a lot of time in our room.

Not long later, my opinion of the place radically changes. Not that it suddenly becomes cleaner, but rather we have a sit-down with the owner.

As we settle with our drinks outside in the shade, the Aboriginals are clearing out. Apparently the owner's rules state that the locals and their vehicles must be off the property by 5:00, whatever it takes to make that happen. A crew of ranch hands will push or tow off any vehicles that remain.

We eat dinner with the station workers and the other guests, and the food is good. The owner is married to a woman from Wenatchee, Washington, so even though that is a six hour drive from us, as far as they're concerned, we're from her "home." The owner's son and business partner was college educated in the United States.

The people here are pleasant; bawdy but kind, and many of the drinks are on the house. They are a family. A propane truck driver, whose regular delivery route is to Ayers Rock, stops in for a meal after an emergency delivery run and has a hard time leaving. This is his family, too. Life here seems pretty good.

Initially, on physical appearance alone, the place made me uncomfortable and I questioned the wisdom of staying here. However, when I took the time to see the inner workings of the place, my impression completely altered. Had I not given the place a chance I would have missed out on a gem of an experience and some of my best memories of the trip.

We can see the night sky horizon to horizon here, with only the station lights to interfere. It is here we see the Southern Cross for the first time, and I'm sure glad we came this way.

One key advantage to being in Australia in the off-season and out in the middle of nowhere is that often we get places to ourselves. As we wind our way along the tortured coastline on the Great Ocean Road, we find a quiet almost undisturbed little beach amongst the cliffs. It has a wooden staircase leading down and no posted signs, but I feel a trespasser in its serenity. There are some human footprints in the sand, but they don't wander far from the bottom of the stairs. The beach sand is red where the rock is red. The exposed cliffs are stained with green algae and white salt. I prefer my beaches this way; wild and empty of other humans, except the one I can hold hands with, or in whose pockets I can shove my frozen fingers. We walk for a ways, further than the previous footprints indicate, but the cold wind and spitting rain make us glad to return to our warm car.

Through winding roads and wine country, we make our way back to Sydney for our final two nights of the trip. I am looking forward to getting home to my cats and dog, to beginning the routine of my new job and especially to married life with Ian. I'll miss Australia, if only for the adventure and the freedom from responsibility it has offered us.

Chapter Forty Six
Learning Curves

But responsibility is what I return home to as I start my new job. I still believe I can make a career in production, and I see this as an opportunity to work with people from whom I can learn. This production team does not produce the boring talking head videos that one associates with government. The projects are creative, interesting, clever and sometimes witty. My new work place has a studio, control room, music library and an edit suite. We have cameras, sound and lighting equipment for shooting on location. The producers have the ability to hire professional talent and extra production staff as needed if budget allows. The state managers invest in keeping the technology up to date.

For me it's a new direction, worth the cut in pay and lack of job security for the chance to grow professionally. I am grateful that Ian's income is enough to support us both if needed and grateful also for his job security.

The expectations are completely different here, and despite my previous training and experience I am overwhelmed, frustrated and terrified by how much I don't know. I have moved from a one-person operation to specializing in editing. I worry that my skills are not what they expected and that they regret hiring me, but I am determined to battle on. I work hard to develop my technical skills to master the equipment, as well as the sense of timing and aesthetics required by an effective editor.

When we upgrade to a strictly computer-based AVID non-linear digital editing system, my steep learning curve becomes a vertical rock face, so I pull out my climbing gear and start the ascent. Non-linear editing opens up new territory for us. Layers of video and audio are manipulated in ways not before possible and are much easier to change. Once I get the hang of it, the old system seems so archaic and I never want to go back.

The following summer, Ian and I buy a house that is approximately two miles from the place we had been renting. It is a log home on 5 acres.

Dancer, my pony, moves with us to our new property, but she is old, has medical issues, and her abilities are limited so now that I have more land, I begin shopping for a riding horse.

In 1992, Breyer released a porcelain model of an Icelandic Horse, which I had quickly added to my ever-growing model horse collection. Now that I'm ready to shop for a horse, I look at my lovely porcelain model, recalling that day I ogled over the information in my breed book, and wonder if anyone in the area sells Icelandics.

I do a web search, which provides only sparse offerings. However, one farm advertising Icelandic horses for sale turns out to only be about an hour away! I can hardly believe it. *Must be fate!*

Icelandic horses are considered to be a gaited breed, which means in addition to the standard three gaits that most horses have which are walk, trot and canter, they generally have a fourth gait called the tolt. It is a four beat gait which is very smooth to ride because the horse has at least one foot on the ground at all times. The comfortable, non-jarring ride and exceptional temperaments are two reasons why the Icelandic horse is desirable. Yet its scarcity makes it expensive to buy.

I can hardly contain my excitement as Ian and I pull up to the riding arena where the owner of these horses has arranged to meet us. In my phone conversations with him, he tells me that he has only untrained horses for sale in my price range but he has one I can ride so I can experience the special gait.

The arena is on a friend's property as they don't have a good place to ride on their family farm. The chill of fall is in the air, and so is the distinct smell of horse manure. It's enough to make you aware of the presence of horses without being overpowering.

The boy who greets us is in his mid-teens and introduces himself as Rex. He leads me over to the horse I will be riding. She's a fuzzy little black mare, standing patiently.

"She seems small," I comment.

"Don't let the size fool you. She's plenty strong," Rex assures. He introduces the mare as Nott.

He puts on a saddle that is different from any I've seen before. It's like an English saddle, only with a flatter seat that is padded and ribbed by lines of stitching. He places it back from the shoulder and girths it up. The bridle is likewise different, consisting of the bit attached to a single strap that goes around the ears. A separate piece rests behind the ears and fastens around the nose in front of the bit. This is called a dropped noseband.

He gets on first, and she surges forward. He lifts his hands and begins a see-saw motion on her mouth with the reins and I see the little mare start to glide into the tolt. Even in the soft arena, I hear the clear four beat gait as she chugs along.

"When you ride her, in order to get the tolt, you need to do like I'm doing with my hands," he says. "Lift your hands, then just a bit of alternating with the reins."

He holds her bridle while I mount. It's not a challenge with a horse whose back is this close to the ground.

"Be sure to keep your legs off her sides," he cautions. "That's her cue to go faster."

I don't know enough to be nervous. I still have my full array of confidence, considering myself a rider with some experience.

I hold my legs a little away from her and she starts forward as soon as Rex lets go of the bridle. She definitely feels larger in the body than her small stature would indicate, and her walk is energetic. The ribbed, padded saddle is comfortable. After a few minutes of walking and getting a feel for her, Rex encourages me to ask her to go faster.

"OK, now lift up your hands and pull back on the reins," he instructs.

As soon as I do this she speeds up. I don't even have to put my leg on her, since she knows that the lifting of the hands is her cue to go forward into the gait. But it's not very smooth like I would expect from the propaganda.

"Alternate pulling with your hands like I showed you," he instructs.

I start the see-saw motion and she lifts her head up and her gait becomes smoother, her long black mane flowing back towards me and tangling between my fingers and the reins. The sound is like a little freight train gliding down the track: tic-ka-ticka-ticka-ticka. It is exhilarating and I am hooked. I don't want to get off.

I would find out later that this style of riding is old fashioned and not considered to be kind to the horse, but at this stage I am almost completely incapable of recognizing such things, including the fact that I am not much of a rider. Nott becomes the first of many Icelandics I will sit astride, marking the beginning of a long educational journey.

Thrilled by this experience and excited at the prospect of owning my own, we arrange to meet where his horses are kept; on his family's small family farm a few miles away.

At his place, one of the first things I notice is that there seem to be a lot of these small fuzzy horses in varying colors in small pens that are devoid of grass.

The horse Rex has in mind for me is a tall chestnut gelding named Rísi, who has turned four this year. This is considered to be the correct age to start his training. Rex goes into the pen where Rísi is contained with several other horses, and immediately Rísi runs away from him. We spend the next ten to twenty minutes watching as Rex tries to walk the horse down. Each time he is approached, Rísi trots away or puts other horses between Rex and himself. The pen may be small, but the horse still has plenty of space to employ his evasive maneuvers successfully for quite some time.

"Um, should he be so hard to catch?" I ask stupidly, tiny alarm bells chiming dully in the recesses of my brain.

"Oh, he'll be fine," assures Rex. "He just hasn't been handled much. He'll come around."

I silence the alarms and stumble trustingly forward. After all, Icelandics are kind, good tempered and brave horses. Of course it will be fine.

So in 1997 I buy my first Icelandic horse. I sell some of my model horses and madly work on restoration projects in order to be able to afford the payments I have arranged. Rex arranges for him to have a couple of months of training at a farm across the state that specializes in Icelandics.

When Rísi comes back, he is still hard to catch but at least he has been started under saddle. However, there are more hard lessons in store for me. I am soon to learn how little I know about riding and how little he knows about being ridden. I pay dearly for my naivety, but my experiences with this horse change the direction of my life.

Rísi and I start having problems almost immediately. My lack of skill means I don't know how to communicate with him properly, which makes him tense and nervous, which in turn makes me tense and nervous. We feed off of each other's nervousness, which can only end in disaster. Eventually he responds by doing what many horses do when they are insecure, afraid and lack leadership- he invokes the flight response. In other words, he bolts.

His brain disconnects as he panics and he runs fast and furious. Terrified, I pull on the reins but to no avail. Deciding that I'd rather control my own fate than risk where he might take me, I bail off onto the hard gravel road. Rolling painfully to my feet, I limp after him. He stops not long after my departure and I am able to catch him and we walk towards home. He is calm now, but I am bruised and badly shaken. After several of these incidents, the damage is done. My confidence is tattered and I become afraid. I have a decision to make: give up or get help. I choose the latter.

I begin to acquire resources; to contact and meet other people who own Icelandic horses. I attend riding and training clinics, learn about establishing leadership through groundwork, and ride, ride, ride in an effort to overcome my fear. I ride Rísi as well as other horses. At first I tense up and pull on the reins every time a horse goes faster than a walk. I have lost my ability to trust. There are many horses who would not even think of taking off with me, but I am apprehensive that any of them might.

Meanwhile, Rísi still bolts. Eventually I learn to ride these out instead of bailing off, but even then I sometimes end up being thrown to the hard ground by a sudden turn or sliding stop.

To add insult to injury, Rísi doesn't have an apptitude for tolt, the smooth gait that I assumed all Icelandics would have. I do not consider him brave and even-tempered either, which is the other highly desired trait of the breed. More accurately, he is not compatible with my current level of knowlege and skill.

Things might be very different between us had we met at a later stage in my development.

Understanding fear has helped me become a better trainer, because I can empathize with riders and their apprehensions. When a horse reacts a certain way, I can comprehend how this can be disconcerting to a less confident rider and I am therefore better able to match people with appropriate horses. So in many respects, I have a lot to thank Rísi for. I definitely would not be where I am now without the rough start he gave me.

Chapter Forty Seven
Career Moves

I love the work I do. I love creating a vision. The projects are extensively overseen by the director, the producer and the client, and I am constantly asked to make changes in the effort to produce a better product. Though this is often a source of frustration for me, ultimately we create some awesome stuff and our projects win numerous awards. If I feel my creative role is significant enough and the award is prestigious enough, I will order my own statuette which I have to do at my own expense. It comes engraved with my name accompanied by the subtext "editor."

Except when we are on deadline and the equipment is acting up, my job offers a laid back and friendly working environment. When I find three 2-week old kittens that had been dropped in the middle of the road to die, I buy formula and begin bottle-feeding them. Their feeding schedule requires that they come to work with me, and everyone pitches in to make sure they get fed. Since Ian and I have four cats already, we cannot keep any of them, but that doesn't turn out to be a problem. Two of the kittens are adopted by co-workers, and the third goes to my sister.

During a private meeting with my boss, she observes that I seem more result oriented than process oriented. She suggests I learn to enjoy the process more.

She has a point. I tend to want to be instantly good at the tasks I take on, craving the destination rather than enjoying the journey. I am impatient for projects to be completed, rather than savoring the creative outlay that makes the work exceptional. While easier said than done, her statement really sticks in my mind and I find myself contemplating it every time I take on a new project or pastime, from my work with horses to learning to play the mandolin.

Since I have taken clinics and worked with instructors to help improve my ability to handle horses, I am beginning to feel like I know something. I am making connections within the Icelandic horse community, and through these I meet up with a woman who has a few Icelandic horses she isn't doing much with. She agrees to let me play with a couple of them at my farm. I do not feel qualified to charge for my work, so initially she pays me only what it costs me to feed them. After awhile, the owner insists on paying me something for my time and effort. I guess she figures that the something I am doing is better than the nothing she'd been doing. Since being paid escalates me from hobbyist to professional, I find myself rather unexpectedly in a second career.

In truth, I don't know much at all. Just when I think I am good at what I do, an instructor, clinician or horse will help me realize how little I know. I come to expect that each time I reach a destination and start to get comfortable, I am presented with another destination further along. It's always my choice whether to buy the bus ticket to the next stop along the route, but with my desire to continuously improve, I usually do.

A couple of years later, my employer loses its state contract. State positions are created for all but editing, which becomes open to pre-approved independent contractors. Most of my co-workers apply for their jobs and become state employees. I have to apply to be on the list of eligible contractors. As with the horse training, I have no idea how to assign an appropriate value to what I do. While I am sure that my value is significantly more than what I was getting from my contract employer, the suggestions regarding what I should be charging seem like a huge jump despite all the extra expenses associated with being self employed. So while my co-workers collect a state paycheck, I learn about submitting work proposals, service agreements, and invoices. Even as I envy their steady hours, income, benefits and increased job security, I appreciate the freedom of freelance work and the flexibility in my working hours.

Of all the projects I am involved with, one series stands out as a personal favorite. We call the project "Little Fox," and it consists of four separate videos for the Department of Social and Health Services on Fetal Alcohol Syndrome. The presentation style emulates Native American story telling, using animals as characters, and each of the four narratives depicts a specific age group: Little Fox is a toddler, Little Mask is a pre-teen raccoon, Sees No Danger is an adolescent bear, and Travels in Circles is a young adult puffin.

The Long House in Shelton is bustling with activity. Cords and wires are strung, lights are positioned, the cameras and monitors are set up, batteries are checked and replaced, costumes are adjusted and make-up applied. The air hums with many voices, some giving direction, some conversing as we wait for the camera to roll. The smell of the natural wood structure blends with lingering incense and more faintly the perfumes and colognes of an assemblage of people. Because of the uniqueness of this production, I've been invited to crew at this distinctive location, so I am among those stringing wires and cables that feed our array of equipment.

Our talent, portraying the Native American storyteller, is actor Floyd "Red Crow" Westerman, decked out in layers of authentic native robes and costuming. Fans of *The X-Files* know Floyd as Navajo code talker Albert Hosteen from the episode

"Anasazi" (season 2, episode 25). Being an *X-Files* fan myself, I'm thrilled to be in the same room with him, but in the interest of maintaining professionalism, I keep my distance.

A small throng has been assembled to make up the storyteller's audience, drawn from the clients, production staff and their families. This gives us a wide range of ages and ethnic groups.

It's a lengthy and grueling shoot. Floyd is reading from a teleprompter yet trying to make it look and sound as if he isn't. The scripts are long and each section requires multiple takes. While Floyd delivers his lines, a second camera grabs a variety of shots of the audience, looking interested and captivated by his stories. These shots allow us to cut away from Floyd during editing to cover places in the narrative where we need to edit two different takes together so he doesn't have to deliver volumes of script flawlessly, as well as allowing us to transition between different angles of Floyd to add visual variety. The final cut for each video is to be 20-30 minutes and even though there will be some dialogue by characters in the stories, this still results in a lot of material for Floyd to convey.

An artist is hired to provide illustrations for each of the stories. These will be cut into the narrative where appropriate to help hold the viewer's interest. Some of the artist's depictions are very good, but his work is inconsistent. I'm told this is due to a substance abuse problem, which is such a shame as he is incredibly talented. His drawings remind me of the progression of British artist William Turner's paintings: the works start out vivid, clean and clear but degrade over his lifetime to practically scribbles on the canvas. This guy manages to produce this same effect over a matter of months and it's not always progressive. For budget reasons we have to accept his work and take the good with the bad.

An intern and I shoot all the artwork in the studio. Many of the animal characters have speaking parts to break up Floyd's narration. Budget constraints mean that we need to use crew and office staff to voice the parts rather than hire professional talent, so we recruit anyone and everyone in and around the office. Eager to contribute, I am given one line, voicing the Octopus in Travels in Circles. The producer seems happy with my read and I am happy that she is happy because I had fun doing it. Less fun is hearing my voice over and over during the edit. Because my face is not camera-friendly, this is the only time I am used as talent during my employment.

By the time we get to editing in the sound effects and music, the project has pretty much fallen into my hands. The rest of the production staff has moved on to other projects. At a producer's recommendation, I obtain permission from a Native American flautist in Seattle to use music from his CDs and his work makes up the majority of the score. We either Foley the sound effects (create them ourselves) or use pre-recorded ones from our library.

As a reward for my efforts, Little Fox wins a Nell Shipman Award for editing excellence from the Seattle chapter of Women in Film. It is the only award that is specifically for my work alone. The series wins a silver Telly, a prestigious industry award, and is nominated for an Emmy after it gets airplay on public television.

Now that I am on call on a per-project basis, I have more time to work with horses. In fact, though I still enjoy editing and it certainly pays better, I am finding that it is starting to get in the way of my horse training as more people seem willing to let me experiment with their animals.

I still have Rísi, but I have purchased two other Icelandics in the meantime. My second Icelandic is a young mare I bought as a yearling from a friend. I plan to raise and train her myself. I wasn't looking for the third horse, a gelding that is a little bit older, but the owner didn't want him anymore and offered him to me at a very good price. Both these horses have the calm, brave dispositions and both show obvious signs of the tolt which is so elusive for Rísi. Though these latter two come to me untrained, their temperaments make them a good deal less hazardous for a novice like me to work with. Since they are more suitable for my level and I can only ride so many horses, I decide that it's time for me and Rísi to part ways. In December of 2000, I sell him to a great home for a fraction of what I paid and never look back, except to ponder my time with him and say "if I knew then what I know now..."

Chapter Forty Eight
The Source

I am totally enamored with the Icelandic horse. When I take on an occupation or a hobby, I jump in with both feet, striving to be the best I can and learning as much as possible as quickly as possible.

I continue to take educational clinics to improve my riding and training skills. I join email groups, which help me connect with Icelandic horse owners, breeders and trainers around the United States, Canada, Europe and Iceland.

I'd chosen a mare as my second Icelandic because I wanted the option of doing some breeding. She's a decent mare, which is pure luck since when I chose her I knew nothing about the breed standards. But now that I know a little more, I want to further enhance my breeding program. I am hoping to find a second mare of even better quality with more proven bloodlines that I can enjoy as a riding horse but also get a foal from now and then. I begin my search in the United States and Canada, but soon realize how fun and educational it could be to go straight to the source. In 2001, I journey to Iceland for the first time, dragging Ian along with me.

I am eager not just to go horse shopping, but to see this beautiful country I've heard so much about. Through my personal and on-line connections and acquaintances, I've arranged to visit several farms with promising horses for sale. My plan is to spend the first week trying horses and visiting people, some of whom I've communicated with but never actually met, and the second week exploring the less-populated eastern side of Iceland, ultimately circling the entire country via the ring road.

I get my first look at the green of Iceland as the plane approaches for landing and the sun is rising. It's been a long trek for us, and even through the fog of exhaustion my stomach flips with excitement. Flights from the United States to Iceland tend to leave in the evening, which means when you add the time difference you are arriving in Iceland around six the following morning. For this particular trek, we flew from Seattle to Baltimore and caught a connecting flight to Iceland, so the combined flights have taken their toll.

There is a misconception that the airport is in Reykjavík, but it is actually in Keflavík, about 30 miles to the southwest. This is near the US military base and is not heavily populated, so instead of landing in a city, we find ourselves in desolate territory. As we emerge from the building, the sky is gray and the air is crisp and breezy, which feels refreshing to our weary senses. The odor is a mix of jet fuel, diesel and salt at this coastal airport. But then, in Iceland, it's difficult to get very far from the coast.

The drive from Keflavík to Reykjavík gives us our first look at the tattered landscape of this volcanic island from ground level. The fields are jagged and rocky with ancient black pillow lava and the soil is dark with smatterings of green moss rather than grass. I can't imagine walking through that landscape, and it is no wonder I don't see horses grazing there, though my eyes scan for them. We've rented a car, which is expensive but it gives us freedom and mobility. I prefer not having to impose on other people for transportation or be enslaved to the uncertain schedules of public transport, especially when I don't speak or read the language.

Our first meal in Iceland is a fish buffet at a pub below the guest house we are staying at in Reykjavík. Fish is a staple of this small island country and they know how to cook it perfectly and with just the right spicing to enhance the flavor. Not all of it is cooked. Some of the options are served raw, and I also choose to overlook the fact that in some cases we have no idea what we are eating.

After visiting some friends in Reykjavík, I've arranged a brief two-day excursion to one of the many farms offering day treks into the country side on horseback. Ian gamely comes along. The first day is a private ride with only Ian, me and the guide, but the scenery is unremarkable. Ian's horse partakes of a slow pounding lateral gait we in the breed refer to as "pig pace." It is not unusual for Icelandic horses to have pace, and it is considered the fifth gait, but it is only correct when done fast and is therefore referred to as "flying pace." Even my horse isn't very comfortable, and I am much relieved that I am offered the opportunity to switch to a delightful little mare with smoothness and energy for the latter part of the ride. It is common to trek with extra horses and she was brought along as the spare.

That evening, Ian complains that his back is sore, but I figure it's just from doing an activity he's not used to. For the longer - and what proves to be more spectacular - ride the next day, I beg for a smoother horse for him and my request is granted. However, by this time the damage has been done.

I visit a number of farms and ride quite a few horses, but a couple of factors are working against me. My confidence is still badly shaken by my negative experiences with Rísi, so I have become a timid rider. Secondly, I discover that I have no idea what I'm looking at. I'm not yet educated enough to recognize a quality horse when I see or experience one.

After driving sixteen kilometers on a rutted but passable gravel road which seems to be getting worse the further we go, we finally arrive at a farm at which is offering some mares for sale. It is nestled in misty hills, dotted with sheep and horses.

We are greeted with typical warm Icelandic hospitality in this idyllic setting. When I eventually get a chance to meet the horses, however, they make me very nervous. The mare which is supposed to be easy turns out to be twitchy and sets me on edge, which doesn't make riding any of the other horses easier since I've become tense and uncertain. Horses in Iceland are encouraged to be forward and energetic, but at this stage of my development their willingness and speed scare me. There are one or two mares I won't even get on as I watch them dance under their rider, difficult to mount and barely in control.

At another farm, a woman shows me a young gray mare. I had specifically requested not to see gray horses, but figuring there has been a communication snafu about this, I decide to go ahead with the ride. If the mare is impressive enough I am willing to consider any options. The woman puts me on what she considers an easy horse while she rides the young mare she intends to show me. The horse I am given is large for an Icelandic, but is considered safe enough for children to ride and which also has easy tolt. However, once the ride begins, I realize I have basically no control over this child's mount. I am just along for the ride, and though it should not be a scary experience I find anxiety creeping back. When I express my concerns to my companion who is riding next to me on the barely-trained little gray mare, she seems surprised and disappointed. If I can't handle the simple horse, there is no way I can handle the horse she is offering for sale. As we return to the barn, my hostess is polite but I get the definite sense from her that she expected me to have better riding skills and that she feels her time has been wasted. Humbled and feeling badly about this, I move on to the next farm.

Two trainers, Magnús Lárusson and Svanný (Svanhildur) Hall, who have made frequent visits to the United States and been very helpful with my struggles with Rísi, are now working at a horse center called Gauksmýri (GOYKS-meer-ie). It is being run as a guest house, so Ian and I rent a room there for a couple of nights so we can socialize and be shown horses for sale.

Gauksmýri also houses working students, so half the building has guest rooms and the other half has student living quarters. The television is nearly always on. We are sitting in the dining area chatting when one of the students rushes in from the other room.

"An airplane just crashed into one of the World Trade Center towers in New York City!" he announces excitedly in excellent English.

The date is September 11.

I don't know what to make of the news. Everyone crowds into the TV room. The news is in Icelandic but the student translates for us so we get the gist of what is going on. The hope for minimal loss of life at the initial impact, the shock as the second plane hits, and the sinking feeling in the pit of my stomach as the towers crumble. Everyone in the room is affected, some even more than us, and we are the only Americans there.

Being out of the country lessens the impact considerably. We certainly are not bombarded with as many intimate details in Iceland and we would have been had we been home, and as a result I am a bit numb to the implications of it all. Even in Iceland, however, it does warrant coverage for a solid 24 hours after the incident. The world is truly watching as offers of aide pour in from all over. Iceland offers a team to help search the rubble but is politely turned down.

Yet despite emails from friends in the States describing the situation and the news coverage, I don't fully appreciate the extent of loss of life and the emotional impact until after we return home. We've been too removed.

Chapter Forty Nine
Silver Linings

Akureyri is our last stop for horse shopping. We have a place to stay in town: the parents of a trainer I know who is attending college in the US are kind enough to let us stay with them. The trainer's friends show me a horse she has for sale, and I visit the stable of another well-known trainer and view a horse there as well.

By the end of the shopping portion of the trip, I've taken photos of each horse and made a few notes, but I am not enthralled by any horse in particular. None jump out at me as being *it*. Several seem like good options, but I have to consider my own riding abilities as well as the needs of the American market. As strong as Icelandic horses generally are, there are many American riders who will be too heavy for a smaller horse to carry comfortably. Perhaps I am being too practical. I'd been hoping that the right horse would make itself somehow obvious, but there is no horse ala *The Black Stallion* that I instantly fall in love with and that falls in love with me.

With visions of the horses I've seen tolting in my head, I will have time to think everything over. We are about to embark on the vacation half of our journey, traveling along the eastern coast, and I'm looking forward to kicking back and relaxing for a bit.

The morning of our departure, however, Ian wakes up with excruciating pain in his lower back. It is so debilitating that he can't move. We take him to the hospital here in Akureyri, which thankfully isn't far from where our hosts live. Meanwhile, our hosts kindly allow me to stay with them while the doctors try to figure out what to do with Ian besides putting him on medication for the pain. The medical staff determines via CT scan that he has a prolapsed disk in his lower back. They suggest that he rest to see if it gets better on its own.

Ian blames the horse trek earlier in our trip. Most likely, however, this is the result of cumulative abuse over a number of years for which a rough ride was the final straw.

My emotions are a mix of concern for him, empathy for the pain he is in, and devastation that the rest of our trip has to be canceled. As much as I'd enjoyed shopping for a horse, I'd been especially looking forward to seeing a different and less populated part of the country with no schedule or obligation except to return to Reykjavik in time for our flight. Now I am left to wonder how we are going to make it home. Due to the chaos caused by 9-11, we are able to postpone our flight a week at no additional charge, but will Ian be OK to travel?

While Ian is laid up, I spend the majority of my time keeping him company, but I also take time for a few sight-seeing excursions. I don't enjoy them nearly as much alone as I would in his company, but these also give me opportunities to contemplate and gather my thoughts.

On one such excursion, I sit alone on the rocks above Goðafoss, or "waterfall of the gods," hearing the roar, feeling the spray and marveling in the awesome power of gravity. There are no barriers, fences, or warning signs, just my own common sense and self-preservation to keep me from venturing too close to the edge. This is so different from any similar location in the United States. The Icelandic government isn't trying to protect me from my own stupidity, and I revel in the sense of responsibility they have given me. Like the cliff above Scarborough, England, this place embeds itself in me and reminds me that I am but a small living creature amidst nature's power. The wind, the roar, the spraying mist of cascading water mixing with hazy drops of rain cold on my face and dampening my hair, the sense of danger from being close to the edge, the dank smell of wet rock and earth as I breathe in; I absorb it all. As if by taking it all in, I can squeeze out my unwanted emotions, tattered by stress, worry and disappointment, throwing them over the falls and leaving me with only serenity and strength.

I also take time to revisit some of the local stables, taking a second look at horses and talking more with the owners and trainers.

After several days Ian is able to travel carefully by car. He is issued crutches and given a prescription for pain pills. The drive back to Reykjavík is only a matter of hours. If Icelanders have to drive an hour, they consider that to be a long distance and a great amount of time. For me, driving from literally one end of the country to the other in four hours is nothing. I can't even drive lengthwise across my own state in that amount of time.

We stay a few days with our friends in Reykjavík. Our hostess is an American, daughter of one of my Icelandic horse mentors. She has been living in Iceland since her late teens and is fluent in the language. She makes a few phone calls and sets up an appointment for me to look at an interesting mare for sale. She comes with me as advisor and translator, and I am grateful for the company and the help.

The mare is solid black and has a large expressive eye and plentiful mane. Otherwise she is nondescript, and it is by no means love at first sight. She's not especially tall, but at least she appears to be sturdy. A rider shows her to me first, and then I ride her myself. There is a lot of power in this mare and I'm not sure how much control I actually have, but the ride goes well enough. I am told that I am a very "kind" rider, when the reality is I have no real clue what to do up there. I fail to appreciate at the time how good this mare really is. Several times during this trip I have been complimented on my riding, which I find very flattering. In hindsight, I realize it probably means they have seen many riders far worse so it is faint praise indeed, as the rider of the gray mare would testify.

This mare's name is Askja, and she's just been evaluated. This means that she has been shown to judges who scored her for conformation (the way she is put together) and for how she goes under saddle including each gait, her willingness to please her rider, and how she carries herself. The higher the score, the closer her qualities are to the breed standard, or ideal Icelandic horse. Her scores are respectable, and even quite good in key areas. This of course affects her price, making her more expensive than I'd originally budgeted.

I make an offer and it is accepted. Buying Askja is a practical decision, not an emotional one, but it is a decision I will never regret. If our vacation plans hadn't changed due to Ian's back troubles, I likely would never have found her.

In the meantime, my friends Magnús and Svanný have made me a proposal on a young untrained mare they have for sale. For what I consider a modest price, they offer me the mare, board for her in Iceland for two years, and the opportunity to come to Gauksmýri for six weeks as a working student at no cost except for what I wish to pay for extra riding lessons. I consider this to be an offer I can't refuse, so instead of one mare I buy two. So it goes.

I manage to get Ian safely home, where he eventually has back surgery and a long recovery.

Meanwhile, my job as a contract editor is gradually dwindling away. The producers are using another contract editor more and more, as well as utilizing internal staff for editing the smaller projects. Eventually they quit calling me at all. I am busier than ever with the horses, so a large part of me doesn't mind.

I allow my contract to lapse and I choose not to pursue editing work elsewhere, since I don't have my own editing system, and my commute to a larger market is impractical.

Thus the Icelandic horses become my full time occupation.

Chapter Fifty
A Part of Something

For the second time in as many years, an Iceland Air plane with me on it touches down in Keflavík.

It is now 2002, and I am completing the transaction with Magnús and Svanný for their young palomino mare. I am excited to have this opportunity to immerse myself in Icelandic culture and training the horses in their native country. My friends have been my instructors and clinicians on many occasions, so I am already familiar with their teaching style and methods. Theirs is a gentler way, which helps build trust and understanding with the horse. My mare is still on the farm and they will guide me through the process of training her.

I've boarded out the three horses I currently own so Ian doesn't have to care for them during the six weeks of my absence. I'll miss Ian terribly, but am grateful to him for being supportive of this opportunity.

The sky is leaden on the fall day of my arrival. Even so, the greens in the pitted fields are vivid and bright. Since I will be in the country for six weeks, I am burdened with several pieces of luggage which I drag with me to customs. Signs are posted, reminding visitors to protect against bringing diseases into Iceland by disinfecting any equipment that has had contact with animals outside of this isolated country. I have done this prior to my departure, but am surprised that no one asks or checks.

No rental car for me this time around. A shuttle runs from the airport to one of the major hotels in Reykjavík. No reservation needed and you pay on board. I have a stash of Icelandic kronur ready for such a purpose.

The combined flights have me pretty wiped out, but I am eager to begin my new adventure. Adrenalin will keep me going for awhile, at least.

Though I was here for only a few weeks the previous year, I am amazed how familiar everything looks. I recognize the names of towns and places as well as landmarks and terristrial features. Perhaps it is because we'd rented a car and did the driving ourselves, which forced me to pay more attention to the details of the roads, landscape and cityscape.

My arrival has been coordinated with other farm business in Reykjavík, so once I arrive there I have a ride to the farm. Iceland has buses that run the ring road, which is the main road that circles the entire country and is appropriately given the number "1." But catching a lift saves me a lot of hassle and expense, for which I am grateful after a long and tiring flight.

The horse center Gauksmýri is owned by Magnús's sister Sigga and her husband Jói. It rests about two hours north and a bit east of Reykjavik, directly off the ring road. The nearest town is Hvammstangi, and Akureyri is two hours to the east. If you travel north from Gauksmýri you'd be on fjords.

Sigga is working hard to make Gauksmýri a guest house, with sleeping accommodation and a full service restaurant. She runs her own small horse breeding program and offers a full service horse training facility as well as horse trekking for guests. There are four main buildings, surrounded by pasture. The dominant building combines the restaurant and guest rooms on one end of the upper storey, with the other end of the house devoted to a common room, laundry room, shower, and sleeping rooms for the working students. The lower storey features self-contained living quarters where Magnús and

Svanný reside. Sigga and Jói have a house adjacent to the main building. For the horses, there is a barn, though few actually live in it. Last but certainly not least is the riding hall, spacious and completely enclosed. In addition to the riding area, it has teaching spaces and viewing areas. By Icelandic standards, this is a lavish facility. It is the off-season, and while we have a few visitors now and again, for the most part we working students have the place to ourselves, except when Sigga hosts special events and parties.

During my brief time in residence, the number of working students ranges between five and seven. At 36, I am the oldest. The others range in age from late teens to mid-twenties. Most are there for three months at least so I am a short-timer by comparison. We earn our keep by helping to care for the horses, and usually the working students have house chores they are responsible for as well.

"Do you want me to help with the housekeeping?" I ask Sigga.

"No, you already know how to run your own household. These young women need to learn how to do these things."

Sigga has obviously never been to my house. However, I am nonetheless happy to be absolved of household duties.

The very night of my arrival, Gauksmýri is hosting a social event in the riding hall. I am treated as a guest here, though I feel guilty since I have only just arrived and haven't had a chance to earn my keep. I offer to help, but am told to just enjoy myself.

The riding hall is cold and I linger near the outskirts of the party, bundled in winter wear and hovering near one of the heaters that has been set out. There are a fair number of guests, maybe 50 or so. There isn't much else to do on an autumn evening away from the city, so the neighbors flock in. A live band is blaring, and the conversation struggles to rise above it. It's all a blur of noise in my jet-lagged brain, especially considering I don't understand a word anyone is saying. I have a little wine which only makes me more tired and less able to focus. There are hardly any chairs, so the best I can manage is to find places to lean when I get too weary to stand.

I hang with the other students when I can find them because they are some of the few faces that are familiar, but they are keeping to themselves and not talking much either. Some of them turn in early.

I get a few strange looks from guests. My odd appearance combined with being a stranger and obvious *útlendingur* (foreigner) make me a bit of a spectacle, but I am not at all offended since I've been expecting it. Plus I am too tired to care. I make very little conversation. What would I say to a complete stranger who may or may not speak English?

My complete inability to make any social connections as well as my fatigue finally convinces me to follow the lead of many of my fellow students and head in for the night. It is an interesting if awkward welcome to Iceland, but at least I am made to feel that I am a part of something and for that I am grateful.

I have arrived just in time for the regional horse round-up, which takes place the next day. Some of the best summer grazing land in Iceland is owned by the government, and farmers are allowed to free-roam their horses and sheep on it. There are no fences and the horses from different owners intermingle. In the fall, the horses are rounded up and sorted so that they go home with their respective owners for the winter. As it happens, I'd been to a similar event during my previous trip. They are quite common and generally well-attended.

A few of the working students are riding to help bring the herd in, and they go with Magnús and the horse trailer which contains their mounts. Sigga drives those of us who are not riding to the sorting pens. This is a large social gathering with a festive atmosphere and locals as well as tourists will travel from one round-up to another to help out, observe, or just for the party. There is a food vendor, and as the alcohol flows, spontaneous singing erupts amongst a small group of men, growing bigger as others join in. It is a good day since there is little rain, but sweaters knit from Icelandic wool abound in colorful patterns on men and women alike.

As the horses are herded in, a group of them is placed in the central circular holding pen. Men go in and look at each horse for marks of ownership, which might be a freeze brand, an ear notch, or a microchip. Once ownership is established, a horse is pushed through a gate into one of a series of pens that line the perimeter of the inner sorting pen.

As I make my way through the crowd, a robust Icelandic woman approaches me, and in heavily accented English she says:

"I saw you last year, yes?" She rattles off the location of previous year's event. Regardless of whether or not I recognize the name of the place, if she says she saw me, I believe her.

I am not surprised at being recognized. If anything, I should be more surprised that she approached me to ask. Icelanders, while incredibly hospitable, can be shy toward strangers, especially foreigners.

In this particular case, I do not mind being recognized. I find it flattering and it is oddly comforting. I suddenly feel less like an outsider.

It also occurs to me that I've been here less than 48 hours and already I've been to two parties.

The other working students are from European countries. We have several Germans, a Swede, a Dane, and later we are joined by an Icelander. I am the only native English speaker, but the common language is English so that is what we all speak to each other.

I would like to learn Icelandic, but learning a language through immersion has its own challenges. You have to understand what is being asked of you in order to be useful as a worker. I would need to be at a different farm for a longer period to master that. Sigga does attempt to teach us all some basic Icelandic, but I learned most of what little I know through my own studies.

Of course the Icelanders converse in Icelandic and the Germans in German. English is a bit awkward for some of them but we all manage to communicate.

Chapter Fifty One
The Cuckoo's Mire

On a typical working day, we are up early for breakfast. As the wheel of the year spins deeper into winter, the days become shorter and shorter, especially as far north as we are in the hemisphere. We make the most of the daylight, and the riding hall has lights.

Breakfast offers toast with cheese to go on it, yogurt, fruit, granola, tomatoes and cucumbers. Often we are on our own, but if there are guests then Sigga or Jói will come to the kitchen and put out the spread. I grow very fond of cheese on toast, but I am unable to duplicate it in the States. The bread is just different somehow. On the mornings when it is just the students, I am treated to repeated and almost daily playing of Jeff Buckley's cheerful and uplifting version of *Hallelujah*. Those who are familiar with the tune know that I'm being sarcastic. It is lovely but haunting, but day after day I am subjected to it, sometimes several times in a row at one sitting until I am sick of it. After I return home, however, I begin to crave it, like a drug, and that song performed by any artist reminds me of Iceland.

After breakfast, we bundle up appropriately because we need to bring the horses in from the field. It doesn't take all of us, so usually two or three of us take turns. The others are in the barn preparing the stalls by cleaning them and dropping in a bit of sawdust for absorption. Icelanders are very sparing with sawdust because most wood products need to be imported. There's that small problem of having all the existing trees on Iceland chopped down centuries ago, and being so close to the latitudinal tree line that the growth rate is extremely slow. It might take 50 years for a tree to grow six feet. There are reforestation projects all over Iceland, including one small grove on Gauksmýri which we jokingly call "the forest." The horses are not allowed there because they would destroy the trees. I suspect there is government subsidy involved.

What do you do if you get lost in a forest in Iceland?

Stand up.

Only a handful of sawdust is sprinkled in each stall.

The horses know the drill, but some days they are more contrary about coming in and it takes a little more time and coordination. But we persevere and the horses are brought to a holding pen.

The training and riding horses that have been out for the night are sorted into the barn and then into stalls. The structure is a former dairy barn, so the stalls are formed of molded concrete about chest high to a man, the walls thick enough to sit on comfortably. For those of us staying behind to clean stalls, we have a CD player for entertainment. The most often played CD is *The Beatles Live at the BBC*, especially disk one of the two disk set. I get quite sick of it too, but yet again I become reminiscent upon my return home and eventually purchase a copy.

Many of the horses which are not being trained or ridden that day are exercised a different way. Mares with foals, lame horses and youngsters are excused, and once sorted out are allowed to return to the field. Those remaining are let 10-20 at a time onto a small outdoor rectangular track. It is fenced on the outside perimeter, but the inside of the track is defined by ropes. Two of us with long lunge whips stand in the middle, one at each end of the inside of the oval. The idea is to keep the group of horses moving steadily, not too fast but not stopping and especially not getting stuck in corners. It's trickier than it sounds, because they don't always bunch up conveniently, and horses need to be encouraged from behind. If a horse perceives you are stepping in front of its path, it will slow or stop and possibly try to turn around. So you may well be encouraging one from behind while stepping in front of another. This not only exercises the horses, but teaches those driving them when and where to apply and remove pressure. Magnús usually oversees us, with plenty of input. Each group of horses, when finished, is allowed to return to the field.

Some days instead of exercising the horses around the small track, we saddle up riding horses and herd the entire group along the riding paths. These paths are wide enough for tractors and fenced on both sides. Gates mark property boundaries, and often gates will come in from the sides directly from the horse fields. These riding roads run between farms, and though it is not uncommon for riders to travel along major roadways which often have wide shoulders for this purpose, this is a little safer and allows a herd of loose horses to come along. Some of us ride in front to open gates as needed, our horses acting as herd leaders, and some ride behind to push the stragglers along.

Such outings are a good opportunity to ride a horse that is just barely under saddle. These young horses may not know much about cues from the leg or the reins, but they will follow the herd and thus become accustomed to carrying a rider away from home. The presence of the other horses makes them feel more secure.

One clear but especially cold day taking the herd down the corridor, we come to a stop. We sit on our horses while the herd mills between us, looking for anything edible and squabbling occasionally. We wait, passing the time with friendly chatter. We wait some more. Moving out in the cold isn't so bad, but soon I can no longer chat because my lips won't function. My idle hands and my feet are aching. I drop my feet out of the stirrups to improve circulation. The parts of our faces sticking out from our scarves are red. I put my scarf over my mouth and nose, the heat of my breath helping to keep my face warm. I shiver uncontrollably under my layers of clothing, including my own thick Icelandic sweater. We get off our horses, and I try walking around on feet I can barely feel. I'm getting annoyed as I have no idea why we've stopped so long and I am bitterly cold. I am one of the riders at the back of the pack, so I have no clear concept of where we are. I am eventually told that we are waiting for Magnús.

Finally, with apologies, Magnús reappears. Apparently we have been waiting all this time at a neighbor's house where Magnús had business, which likely turned into coffee and conversation. I don't thaw completely out the rest of that day, despite the infusion of warm beverages and a hot shower. Iceland helps me understand the phrase "chilled to the bone."

Weather does play a factor in our work and activities. On days when the wind blows us sideways and the horizontal rain blinds us and creates ponds at our feet while we watch, or when the slanting snow renders visibility to nil, we stay inside and watch movies. Sometimes on those days, Magnús will teach class, usually on conformation and the biomechanics of the horse.

In one particular blizzard, I and one of the other girls volunteer to go out and fetch two stallions from one of the fields. While stereotypes exist of stallions as being aggressive, testosterone-ridden and potentially dangerous, this generally isn't the case with Icelandic stallions. Icelandic stallions are handled, socialized, and are expected to respect humans as much as any mare or gelding would, if not more so. But one of the stallions, a smaller one with a Napoleon complex, has a reputation for being a little evasive. And it's a roomy field.

I'm given the easy one. Thankfully he is dark colored, because in the cascading snow I am looking for a dark horse in a white field. We have to put our heads down and struggle for each step against the wind and piling snow. Tall for an Icelandic and sturdily built, Fönix waits for us once he realizes we are there and willingly allows us to slip on the halter. I think he's just as glad to get out of that crap as we are. The other little bugger, however, takes off and my unfortunate companion must trudge after him. Fönix and I wait, and I track her progress as best I can. I will not leave her in these elements alone, but once I see she has captured her quarry, Fönix and I trek toward the barn. Having the wind at my back pushing is almost as bad as fighting my way into it. It wants to rush me along recklessly through deep snow and over hidden obstacles, threatening to shove me on my face if I put up too much resistance.

A stall in an area separate from the mares awaits each of the boys, and a toasty house and a hot beverage await me and my companion.

Icelanders keep their houses warm. Energy is a commodity on Iceland, so much so that they export much of what they don't use to Europe. Since they are a people living in what can be a harsh climate, I suspect they have come to value warmth. It can be quite the shock walking inside from below freezing temperatures, bundled in four layers of clothing including hat, scarf, heavy gloves, long underwear, an Icelandic wool sweater, a waterproof wind-resistant outer shell and heavily lined boots. You can't peel the layers off fast enough.

Each day after the horses are brought in and before work begins, we have "coffee," which is the generic term for a break featuring a hot beverage and some sort of snack like cake or cookies. They all think I'm odd for not drinking coffee. In fact, I don't drink caffeine at all but fortunately there is herbal tea and on rare occasions hot cocoa. We sit in a heated room in the barn and Magnús gives us the plan and assignments for the day. Sometimes we are left on our own for awhile.

"So do any of you know what "Gauksmýri" means in English?" I ask my fellow students on a day when it is only us.

"Gaukur is cuckoo," one replies.

"And mýri is swamp," another adds.

"Yes," I agree. "Literally translated it would be 'cuckoo's mire.' Maybe cuckoo's nest. Does anyone know what significance that has in American English?"

"Isn't a cuckoo a bird that puts its eggs into another bird's nest?" Someone guesses.

"Yes, but in America, a cuckoo's nest is another name for an insane asylum."

Laughter.

"What does that mean, sane…silum?" asks one who's English isn't as good.

"A place for crazy people."

More laughter.

"Yes that is true!" exclaims one of the Germans. "We are all a bunch of crazy people!"

Chapter Fifty Two
An Education

Mixed in with the daily routine of training, I take private riding instruction from Magnús. Sometimes we ride together down the trail, and sometimes we are in the riding hall.

Magnús has good English and a potentially very loud voice. This leads him to believe that he can shout over almost any other noise. For the most part, he is right.

I've had Magnús as an instructor enough by this time that I am used to him yelling at me. While I take it as an indication that something I am doing needs to change, it no longer upsets me. Frustrates me, perhaps, if I cannot figure out what change needs to be made. The best thing to do in that case is simply ask him what I'm supposed to be doing.

"Ég skilja ekki." I'd say in one of my few Icelandic phrases. *I don't understand.*

But if the rain is pounding on the roof and the wind is doing its best to topple the walls, Magnús's booming voice is lost like a cell phone ringing at a rock concert. Or it echoes off the walls and blends like so much white noise with the storm that the words are unintelligible. It doesn't help that I am nearly deaf in one ear, so if I am circling counterclockwise I have to turn my head his direction.

"Ég heyra þig ekki." *I cannot hear you.*

Of course I don't need to speak Icelandic and usually don't, but it is fun to exercise what little I know.

On one occasion, Magnús asks me to come with him on a ride. I am to ride my young mare and Magnús is taking one of his training horses. At one point, I practice a transition from walk to trot. I hear a noise behind me and turn in time to see Magnús picking himself up off the ground and a very nervous horse dancing around him. I ride back over to a lecture on watching out for fellow riders and not leaving someone behind who is on a nervous horse. I feel terrible. I should have been watching out for him. Yet I had believed I was the one on the young insecure horse. Apparently in this case my horse was the calm one.

Sometimes we have group instruction, which might be in a classroom in the form of lecture with illustrations or in the riding hall working with the horses. Magnús and Svanný both are certified breeding judges, which means they know the characteristics that make up the ideal Icelandic Horse according to the breed standards. We have instruction on breaking down and scoring the conformation and movements of the horses, which I find especially interesting. While it is doubtful I will ever become a breeding judge, it is an area in which I choose to build my knowledge as much as practically possible.

Gauksmýri is the center of my world in Iceland, but thankfully I am not confined to the farm, or even restricted by how far I can get on horseback.

Since I know Magnús and Svanný on a social level and consider them friends, sometimes I am invited to go with them on trips. I enjoy getting off the farm and seeing the country. On one excursion, they take me with them to look at young horses on another farm, and we hike far into the field. There is much discussion and young horses are encouraged to move so that their gaits can be watched. How a horse moves is more important in Iceland than how it looks. Icelanders like energy, high leg lift, and long reaching strides. The body should be free, flexible and supple rather than stiff. But I am not yet any good at recognizing these traits, so I can only stand back and observe and wait, trying not to get too cold. I cannot help getting wet, since it is raining. It often is in Iceland. If Icelanders let rain stop them from doing anything, they'd never get anything done.

Some trips we stop at someone's house, either because they are friends, they have business, or both. Icelanders are very hospitable. They always have coffee and some sort of food like cake or cookies for their guests. And they talk, often for long periods of time. Or maybe it seems like long periods of time because I can't hardly understand anything they say.

Not that I haven't made some effort to try. People are impressed when I say to them "Ég er að læra islensk." *I am learning Icelandic.* My grasp of the language remains only rudimentary. It is a difficult language anyway, but without immersion, it is nearly impossible. In America, I have no interaction. I learn some words like numbers and the days of the week by making up flash cards, but like any language it follows the "use it or lose it" rule. I successfully ordered two hot dogs in Icelandic once but got a whole sentence back in Icelandic and had to confess I didn't understand a word of it. "Ensku?" I had to ask sheepishly. *English?*

If the discussion is about horses, I can follow a little. I can recognize horse names and the names of farms. But my vocabulary isn't good. I can understand written Icelandic better than I can write it, write it better than I can speak it providing I have dictionaries and time, and speak it better than I can hear it. Nevertheless by the time I leave Iceland, I can separate and recognize words, even if I don't always understand what those words mean, rather than hearing the words blurring together as unfamiliar sounds.

Sigga and Jói have an old Subaru that students of driving age can sometimes borrow. I am allowed to take it on a couple of trips, including one to Akureyri where I visit the couple with whom I'd stayed the previous year while Ian was in the hospital. I learn the hard way that you don't fill up the gas tank in Iceland. Paying around $100 to fill the tank on a relatively small car is sticker shock indeed.

For one excursion, I catch the bus and have it drop me in Varmahlíð, where an acquaintance picks me up so I can visit her farm on the northern tip of Skagafjörður. She graciously allows me to spend the night there. In her living room I watch *Shrek* dubbed in Icelandic with English subtitles, and I peruse the children's picture books in an effort to improve my Icelandic vocabulary. My hostess finds this amusing, but admits that this is how children learn the language.

Unable to sleep, I take a midnight stroll into the frozen air, eager to see if the sky will put on a show for me. I drift briskly through the cluster of buildings so that their mercury vapor lights don't interfere with my view of the sky. I find myself on the road. I have no light with me, so I have only what moonlight there is and the feel of the ground beneath my feet. The dirt and mud are frozen solid and there has been snow, so I need to be careful not to slip on ice or trip over unseen ruts and obstacles. Glances at the sky as I make my way along indicate that I am not to be disappointed. The road is fairly smooth and clear, and I wander up a ways until the beacons of the buildings are visible but distant. Aurora Borealis, or northern lights, are a common sight especially in Iceland's dark winter sky, but from Gauksmýri I haven't witnessed a spectacle with such color, intensity and activity. At the farm they always seem so distant, monochrome and somewhat stagnant. Here, I am treated to vivid displays of green and blue dancing and waving in a curtain across the star field of a clear black sky. Tired of straining my neck by looking upwards, I lay down flat on my back in the cold hard road, figuring since everything is frozen solid

I'll be less likely to get dirty. I lay there for awhile, taking it in, watching the charged particles of the solar wind weave bright patterns in the Earth's ionosphere. I hear movement near me and sit up, turning my head. In a moment I identify the rustling and crunching to be a small herd of horses moving on the other side of the fence. I hear the occasional familiar snort of a sneeze. I cannot see them, but am acutely aware of them with me in the darkness.

I think of Ian, as I've done many times on this trip. I wish he was here with me, lying there on the solidified mud looking up at the brilliant sky, though I'm not sure his back could take it. I've talked to him at least weekly since I've been gone, but it's no substitute for his company.

The hardness of the ground and the bitter cold take their toll, and I rise. I find my way back to the lights of the quiet, warm house, sliding as quietly as I can into the bed they have prepared for me.

Chapter Fifty Three
An American in Iceland

Since I have a high metabolism and burn energy, one of my favorite topics is food. Lunch is the main meal at the farm, and except on weekends we have a cook who prepares it for us, and she is a good cook. Fish is common, and she finds a variety of ways to prepare it. She is adept at spicing and there's always plenty so that we usually have leftovers. I'm not always keen on the menu choices, but I never go hungry. One dish served fairly regularly are meatballs in white sauce. The meatballs come frozen in a package, and are referred to by the working students as "mystery meatballs." I've never been a huge fan of meatballs anyway, and even less so with white sauce, but they are palatable enough when there are no other options and I'm hungry from working all morning. I suspect they have a variety of different meats in them, including sheep and possibly horse.

Icelanders eat horsemeat, and I'm totally fine with that. Not that it matters to them what I or any other American thinks. Yes I love horses. I love their feel, smell, attitude, interaction, curiosity, and power. But sometimes I don't mind them in a stir fry with ground black pepper and red wine sauce over rice. Svanný cooked such a meal for me once and I quite enjoyed it. Often even Icelanders don't eat horses they've raised themselves. Instead, they trade with a neighbor. However, there are one or two horses we work with on the farm that I would not mind eating. Heck, there are horses I've worked with here in the States I would not mind eating. Breeders of horses in Iceland have the advantage of being able to eat their mistakes. Bad temperament, poor gaits, inability to reproduce, debilitating conformation flaws, dangerous to people; any of these traits can put a horse on the dinner table. Thus these individuals are eliminated from the gene pool.

My motto when it comes to food is that I'll try anything once as long as it won't kill me, and I have several opportunities to follow through. I haven't had the pleasure of trying kæstur hákarl, (fermented shark), but I am treated to a few other cultural delights. One day, as a special treat, we are served sheeps head, complete with eyes.

"We don't eat the brains anymore, because of the mad cow," informs Magnús. I am not disappointed about missing out.

Pulling the meat from the skull is not that different from doing so on any other part of an animal. Some bits are tough and stringy, and I leave those. I can only chew food on one side of my mouth, so anything too leathery becomes an arduous chore. The most challenging aspect is getting enough meat off one head to make a proper meal.

The eye is still in the socket, but it has shrunken some from being cooked. It doesn't look at me. It is glazed over, again from the cooking, so it's not like I'm being stared at while I eat. The eye is considered a delicacy, though I and my fellow students have a hard time seeing it that way. In fact, many of my fellow students have a hard time eating anything from the head at all, opting for the side dishes instead.

It feels somehow wrong, digging the eye out of its socket. This makes me feel more squeamish than the idea of actually eating it. Once I've managed the task, I pop the eye into my mouth.

It's a texture thing. Doesn't have much flavor of its own. Doesn't melt in my mouth, but it squishes between my teeth like jell-o. Even if I am able to get past the notion that I am eating an eyeball, it still feels strange between my teeth. But I chew, swallow, and opt out of eating the second one. Magnús is happy to take care of it for me.

The meat from the uneaten sheep heads is later pulled and made into a loaf for another meal. In this form, however, I am unable to pick out the chewy bits. Muscle and gristle are all contained in this loaf amidst the meaty edible pieces. Even with gravy, it's too chewy and unappealing. I eat very little of it.

Another dish I sample but don't care for is blood pudding. Despite the seasonings, the rich metallic taste is not to my liking. Vampire wanna-bes, this is a dish for you.

I do enjoy Icelandic hot dogs. I don't care how or with what hot dogs are made. I like them anyway. Icelandic hot dogs have a unique flavor, probably from the inclusion of lamb meat, and the sauces and crisp onions typically used as toppings add to the experience.

At a festive community shin-dig at Gauksmyri, one of the dishes served is smoked foal meat. There is quite a bit of breeding done specifically for slaughter, so not all the horses that wind up on the dinner table are culls. I have a bit more reservation about eating foal than I do adult horse, but I go ahead and give it a try. Smoked foal has a rich flavor and, like veal, is very tender.

Unless it is a special occasion, our evening meal is usually leftovers from lunch or whatever else we can scrounge from the fridge. We sit in the darkened dining room, a single light illuminating where we've chosen to sit. After a party, the leftovers are quite tasty and can provide our evening meals for several days. Lucky for us, Sigga knows how to entertain!

It is during one of those dinners early in my stay in a mostly darkened dining hall that I make a non-complimentary comment about President George W. Bush. The girls stare at me incredulously.

"You don't like Bush?" one asks.

"Not particularly," I reply.

"But we thought all Americans like Bush."

"Yeah, you all voted for him!"

"We didn't all vote for him. In fact, less than half of us did."

"Oh."

"Many of us don't like him either."

"He is not so popular with us in Europe."

"No, I don't imagine he would be."

I think they have new respect for me after that. And it makes me realize that the information they get about what's going on in the United States is just as limited as ours is about what's going on in Europe. Propaganda works many ways.

Iceland in winter is beautiful. On trips I take with Magnús and Svanný, I marvel at the scenery when I have daylight enough to see it. The land is criss-crossed with many rivers and streams, forming waterfalls as they spill to lower ground. With late autumn temperatures falling well below freezing, smaller waterfalls are literally stopped cold, turned to ice along with the streams that feed it. These ice-sculptures litter the landscape.

When my stay ends at Gauksmýri and it is time for me to return to Reykjavík, Magnús again drives me. I will stay with my friend in the city until departing for my flight in Keflavík. We pass through a familiar valley, now white with snow.

"It's quite lovely," I comment.

"This is the only time of year that it is lovely," he replies. "Usually it is ugly."

He's right. Normally this is a brown expanse of dirt and rock. The uniform unblemished snow blanket veils this.

Magnús drops me in Reykjavík, and I say my farewells.

As the bus takes me toward Keflavík and ultimately home, I reflect on what I've learned. I have pages of notes which I may never read again, but the act of writing them down helps me retain the information.

My life has been changed, but I cannot exactly express how.

Despite primarily speaking my native language, I have been immersed in another culture. My focus has been horses, with few other distractions. I have eaten their food, been a guest in their houses, driven their roads, and spent their currency. I have visited their country without being a tourist. Rather, a student at age 36, working alongside, learning with and learning from students nearly half my age from several countries. How can this not change you? Interacting with another American has been a rarity. And you know what? I am fine with that.

But I'm just as fine with going home to my husband, my pets and my horses.

Chapter Fifty Four
Humble Pie

For me, vanity is not attached to my appearance, but rather to my performance. But humble pie, while not easy to swallow, can nonetheless be very nutritious.

Five and a half years after my studies in Iceland, I am invited to participate in an educational opportunity for Icelandic horse trainers.

It is a trainer certification course based on the German system, called FEIF Level One, or FEIF Level C. "FEIF" is the International Federation of Icelandic Horse Associations. The acronym comes from the original German name: Föderation Europäischer Islandpferde Freunde, translated literally as "European Federation of Icelandic Horse Friends." The farm hosting the event manages to line up legendary German trainer Walter Feldman, Jr. to instruct the course.

My thinking going into this is *what a great opportunity to get certified for something I already do*. I seem to do decent work training Icelandic horses and my customers are happy, but I've felt for a long time that I don't get much recognition, so I am hopeful that adding credentials will give me additional credibility. I do not expect to vastly improve my training skills in this two-week course, but having some experience as a trainer already should help qualify me.

How hard can it be?

Very hard, as it turns out.

Eight of us are taking the course. We have gathered from all over the country: Washington, New York, Massachusetts,

Georgia, Vermont, and Alaska. In truth, we are guinea pigs. Nothing like this for the Icelandic horse has yet been tried in North America.

On the first day, Walter assesses our riding. I have shipped my mare Thoka to the farm so I have my own horse to ride in the clinic. We are each given comments on the spot, but we are also videotaped for the class to review. I come into this thinking I'm a decent rider. Apparently I am in for a reality check!

We sit around a large television, playing back the tape that shows each of us riding. It is easy to be objective and comment on the positives and negatives of each rider. In large part because of my appearance, I do not take joy in seeing myself on video or in photos, but I understand that video is a great educational tool for objectively showing me what I cannot see from the back of the horse. But in this instance, as I watch myself ride on this video, my face is the least of my worries. I can see for myself that my posture and alignment are all wrong, and I am humiliated. I certainly don't feel all slouchy when I am on the horse, but that is how I appear. My heart sinks and the color drains from my face, I realize that if I am to succeed in this course, I have my work cut out for me. And so does Walter.

The intensity of the curriculum reminds me of being in college, only I seem to have less free time. We are in class from 9-6 daily including weekends, with Sundays being half days, plus there is homework, studying, and we need to practice what we are learning since we have patterns to memorize for the tests.

One gray afternoon several days later, Walter and I are left alone at the dressage ring. Walter is of average height. I am guessing he's in his 60's and he is slightly on the heavier side. He is stout enough that when combined with the white beard evenly framing his face and his round spectacles he might make a decent department store Santa Claus. He wears full seat riding breeches, worn leather boots, a winter jacket, and a baseball cap. The overcast of the day means I can see his eyes behind his glasses. While his authority is absolute, he is nonetheless approachable.

"Walter," I ask hesitantly.

"Yes?"

"How do we compare to groups you've taught in Europe?" I ask.

It is a courageous question, and one I'm not entirely sure I want an answer to.

For me, the anxiety attacks have already begun. We had been informed on the first day of the course that we will have to pass ten tests: gait riding (walk, trot, tolt and canter), dressage, ground work, ponying (riding one horse while leading another) or lunging (moving the horse around you on a line) to be determined by lottery, signal riding, a trail obstacle course, gait theory, teaching, teaching theory, and each of us has to give an oral report. This curriculum is much more advanced than I'd imagined. But with no materials available in English, it had been difficult to relay the expectations of the course in advance to the intended participants.

To give an example of the complexity of the course, take lunging. The trainer moves the horse in a circle around her using a rope attached to its halter. Sounds simple, right? We are using a 50' round pen so the circle is pre-defined and there's nowhere for the horse to go. But everything has to be just so. We are to be judged on the way we carry the whip on approach, how we lead our horse, how we pass through the gate, how our horse passes through the gate, how we hold the whip, how we stand, where we stand, how big the loops in the coiled rope are, how much slack is in the line, the way we use our body, how we use the whip, when we use the whip, how we transfer the whip from one hand to the other, how we ask the horse to go the other direction, how we stop the horse…and the pattern is predetermined so we have to remember that too. And there is a horse in the end of the line, and it doesn't always cooperate, so we have to fix things while trying to maintain composure.

Walter struggles to find the right words to say in English to answer my question. With two native Germans in the group, both of whom have been living in the US for quite some time and whom are quite fluent in English, translating isn't usually an issue. But here it is just the two of us.

"In Germany, riders must have achieved their Silver Riding Badge to be able to participate in this course," he replies thoughtfully. "I don't think this program exists in America yet."

I have heard of the riding badge program, but it is only in the developmental stages for Icelandic horse riders in this country. Loosely translated, what he is saying is that in Germany there is an assumed base of knowledge, like a prerequisite for a college course. We in America are coming at it from all different levels and teaching influences with no proof of prior experience and no expectation for type and level of knowledge.

"And the horses," he continues. "Usually for this sort of course they are better trained."

We have a few well trained horses, but I admit many of them, including my own, are lacking advanced training.

"It is easier for the rider," he adds "if the horse knows everything already."

The bottom line is that several of us may not be up to the proper riding level and some of our riding horses lack adequate training. My thoughts border on despair and I turn away from him, fighting back tears. But qualified or not, I am here and I have no option but to press gamely on.

The mix and flexibility of the curriculum allow us to use time productively regardless of the weather. In light misty rain, hot sun, and even blowing powdery snow we are outside riding, watching Walter give demonstrations, or practicing for the tests.

When the semi-tropical southern rain pounds the red dirt into mud and runs rivulets along the roads and pathways, we listen to hours of lecture on the five gaits of the Icelandic horse, including order of footfall, variations in gait, and how to fix faults in each gait.

To Walter's credit, he brings each of us along to the best of his ability, and ours. If he thinks the horse we are riding absolutely will not work for passing the tests, he says so, but the final decision on which horse we ride in each test is ours. He is a fabulous instructor. His presentation style is no-nonsense, firm and clear. His feedback is good, and we commonly hear "it's OK," "doesn't matter" and "good so" in his thick German accent as he comments on our performance.

Chapter Fifty Five
Moments of Truth

Sleep becomes more difficult the closer we get to test day. I practice what I can when I can with my horse, but time is tight and other people are sharing the space for their own preparations.

The day before the judged tests, we have a full rehearsal. I have committed the patterns to memory and though I know my skills aren't perfect, I have come as far as I can. Thoka works her heart out for me, so I know at least I have a good partner. I have been complimented by both Walter and some of my classmates on how much improvement I've shown in such a short amount of time. I have renewed hope that maybe the goal is not unobtainable after all.

After our run-through, we set about cleaning our tack and equipment and bathing our horses. I pour the whitening shampoo on Thoka, who is now discolored by the crimson clay inherent to the area. When I finish the final rinse, what should be her snowy white mane and tail are now a slight pinkish orange and her dappled brownish gray coat is only tinged slightly red.

The tests are scored on a scale of 1 to 6, with 1 being perfect and 6 being poor to non-existent. We need a score of 4 or better to pass, and we must achieve a passing score on all ten tests in order to qualify for trainer certification. On the plus side, if someone fails any of the tests, they need only retake the ones they fail.

A qualified judge is flown in just for the testing. Walter works with her and may advise her, but ultimately the scoring is up to her. She has no history with us and no preconception, and we do not even meet her until test day.

With butterflies in my stomach, I perform each test. Thoka behaves badly during the lunging test, and I do my best to correct her and keep to the pattern. However, she faces most of the trail obstacles bravely and I swell with pride. While not feeling like any of the tests went perfectly, at the end of the day I come away feeling like I have a shot at passing.

We are not told our scores until the next day. We are called in to face the judges one at a time. Most of those going in before me emerge joyous, and I celebrate their victory as I anxiously await my turn. When my name is called, my heart skips a beat and I go boldly in, optimistic of a favorable outcome.

"Hello, Dawn," the judge greets.

"Hi," I respond, heart pounding.

"I'm sorry to inform you that you did not pass," she continues.

A wave of disappointment and shock pass through me and for an instant I can only stare.

"What did I fail?" I stammer.

"The gait test," she responds, and proceeds to tell me the reasons.

The gait test was the first test. However, I've managed to pass all other nine tests. Through my grief, I am nonetheless relieved that I was not informed of my failure directly after the test, as it might have colored my performance in all the subsequent ones. Some of the tests I barely eek out a passing score, but a pass is a pass.

I try to accept my failure with grace, but I am devastated. I feel like I've let not only myself down but those who helped and supported me along the way.

An opportunity to retake the test presents itself in May of the same year. I invest in lessons, but the effort proves inadequate as I am once again faced with the bitter disappointment of failure. It is obvious that my skills are not where they need to be, but at least this time the judge presents me with a much clearer idea of what skills I need to develop.

Failing the test twice, while a bitter pill to swallow, ultimately proves the best thing for my professional development. Determined not to give up, in July of 2008 I find a dressage instructor not too far from me. The purpose of dressage is to develop and maximize the athletic ability, willingness and responsiveness of the horse and to increase communication between horse and rider. For my part, I need to learn how to relax and how to use my body better, improving my balance and posture while developing more effective and subtle use of my hands, arms, seat and legs.

Had I passed every test, no matter by how small a margin, I might have found myself stuck in a rut. Failure forces me to invest in my continuing education. I am determined that I will pass that test and earn my certification.

On a damp March day of 2010 as the rain threatens but holds back, two borrowed horses take turns carrying me around the same track where I'd failed this gait test twice before. Two years of lessons have prepared me physically for this, and two intense days of private instruction at the farm have prepared me mentally and found compatible horses for me to ride. Still, my heart pounds as I do my best to sit up tall, proud and confident, changing the gaits on cue. A squeeze of one hand, a quick half-halt with my seat, or a touch with my thigh adjusts the movement of the horse, keeping the gait clean and consistent. Canter has been my downfall in the past, and when the judge calls for it my heart skips and I take in my breath, reminding myself to breathe out again. I squeeze the outside rein, cue with the inside leg so the horse picks up the correct lead, and relax back onto the saddle scooping under with my hips to keep my butt in contact and rolling with the horse rather than bouncing off with the rocking movement.

Nervous and breathless, I stand before the judge on the little black mare after the second ride.

The smiles tell me result before the spoken word shares the good news.

"Congratulations, you are now a Level C trainer."

I am filled with relief and elation, and feel a great burden lift from me. Now I have a reason to celebrate.

My education hasn't stopped here. I still take lessons in order to continue to improve my riding, which translates to improvements in my training skills as well. As I become more flexible and balanced, it is easier for me to help the horses I ride become more flexible and balanced. Education is never-ending.

The brush causes a dust cloud as I run it along Thoka's short dappled summer coat. She stands patiently, enjoying the attention, her head and ears in neutral position and her lower lip slack and slightly forward. The fine hairs of her long, thick snow white mane have tangled again, and I'll have to pull apart the snarls by hand. She smells sweet and musky, if slightly like dried manure. I enjoy my relationship with her and each individual horse here, though I could definitely stand to have a few less. While other horse breeds have infiltrated my farm in the past, I am happiest when the population is pure Icelandic.

Feeding Thoka and the other horses gets me out of bed in the morning. While the work can be overwhelming at times, I do some of my best thinking during horse chores, and that work along with riding keeps me active. I primarily train my own horses now, and dabble in breeding a mare now and then. Though the level of my involvement with the Icelandic horse community and other horse-related events may vary, I anticipate these creatures being part of my life in one capacity or another for a long time to come.

Chapter Fifty Six
Being Unforgettable

While I spent my grade school years craving to blend in, as an adult I find more and more reasons to want to stand out.

However, I get uncomfortable when people stare at me. When I take my horses to promotional events where I need to greet the public and answer questions, I get so many curious looks that sometimes I wonder who is actually on display; the horses or me.

I don't mind attention, but I'd rather have it because people are interested in what I have to say or because they like me. Sometimes I pull the pin on my personality and toss it out there like a grenade, with mixed results.

Some are unimpressed. The woman with the asymmetrical face trying to act smart. Trying to grab attention. Trying to be funny. Trying too hard.

Some I win over. If they are interested enough in what I have to say. If I succeed in imparting my knowledge intelligently. If my wit is working. If my authenticity shows through.

If I hide silently in a corner with only my visage as my front, people would notice me in passing, feel sorry for me, then forget me, like the shy piteous figure of Laura with her delicate *Glass Menagerie*, hiding away from the rest of the world. I became determined never to be like that.

But one thing is undeniable. I do get noticed. And sometimes I can use that to my advantage.

I've recently discovered a whole new world of live music. These are bands and artists who make music their livelihood and have a following but are neither rich nor household names. They are restricted by audience size to smaller venues and barely eke out a living, performing out of passion and dedication. I've taken an interest in several of these and I do what I can to support them.

My current favorite is a hard working band out of Virginia called Carbon Leaf. Their song *"The Boxer"* grabbed my attention in 2004 when it got airplay on a Seattle radio station and I became interested in hearing more. Their music is upbeat yet there is a melancholy edge to the message. In general, the lyrics are brilliant, complicated and diverse and the songs are well executed with talent and complexity. Their style is hard to peg, encompassing elements of Celtic, country, folk and rock. Emotionally and intellectually, their music moves me.

Ian and I attend our first Carbon Leaf show in 2005. Most of the songs I am hearing for the first time, and while I enjoy the performance, I can't say that I am totally taken in. But I still like them.

The band announces that they will greet fans after the show, but we are not compelled to stay. The line is long and we have a lengthy drive home. Besides, I have no clue what I'd say to them. I do, however, purchase their latest CD *Indian Summer*. It serves to enhance my appreciation of the band all the more, and remains my favorite of their discography.

Ian is less impressed, but in 2007 I am able to drag him to a second show. We don't meet the band this time either, because they are on a tight schedule and must fly out shortly after their encore.

I buy tickets to see our third show for June of 2009 at the Showbox, a renowned nightclub in downtown Seattle. I learn from their web site that the band will be making a scheduled appearance at a record store near the Seattle Center a few hours before the evening performance. By this time, I've caught up on most of their CD library and consider myself a full-fledged fan. I am enthralled with the possibility of seeing them in a more intimate setting and decide that we're going to check them out.

I have no idea what to expect from their in-store appearance. I don't know if they are performing or just meeting fans and signing autographs. I also have no idea how many people will be attending. I know they have a following in Seattle but I have no concept how large a following it is. Once we arrive, I discover that the band will be performing a short set on a small stage in the back of the store. With minimal lighting and a simple sound system, they play five unplugged songs. No blaring electric guitars and the drummer taps the beat on a single drum. It is so entertaining I worry that it will outshine the performance later that night! More significantly, there are only about 100 people in attendance. Most of the concerts I've attended previously are rock superstars in large venues such as stadiums or amphitheaters, so I'm not used to seeing a favorite band in such small company.

Afterwards, they stick around to talk to the fans and sign autographs. I deliberately move to the front of the store during the last song of the set so I can be first in line. Ian and a friend whom I'd brought along with us are not interested in meeting the band, so my thinking is that I will get the inset of *Indian Summer* autographed and we will have plenty of time to grab a bite to eat and get back downtown to the Showbox before they take the stage.

I try not to idolize people, but I find myself seeking a connection with those whose work I admire. I've tried to rationalize it and I can't find any good explanation. I'm sure that psychological studies have been done and dissertations have been written on the subject, but the bottom line from a layman is people get a thrill and a sense of importance from being close to or being noticed by someone they admire. Even better if that person has reached some level of notoriety. Though I am somewhat ashamed of it, I am no exception. The object of my admiration is Barry Privett, the lyricist and lead singer for the band.

My heart is racing as the band members walk through the store and take positions behind the front counter. I am nervous and I can't diminish the giddiness no matter how hard I try.

I am shortly allowed to approach the band. Barry seems pre-occupied, so I start with Terry, one of the guitarists. I'm not good with faces, but I recognize him because he's a big guy with distinguishable long curly hair. I'd been up close on his side of the stage during the 2007 concert and had caught a wristband he'd tossed into the audience.

"I know it's been awhile, and it's hard to see from the stage with lights in your eyes, but do you remember me from Marymoor a couple of years ago?"

"Oh, sure," he replies. He asks my name and makes his signature mark on the CD inset for *Indian Summer*.

Is he politely giving me the answer he thinks I want to hear? After all, it's been two years, and he's seen hundreds if not thousands of faces at show after show, city after city, venue after venue in the meantime. I hadn't done anything particularly notable that show except catch the wristband. As identifiable as I am, he has no reason to remember me. But I did make eye contact with him, so it is possible that he is telling me the truth.

Terry hands the paper off to Barry, so I turn my attention to him.

"Hi, Barry. I'm Dawn, the one who emailed you about *A Girl and Her Horse*."

"Oh, yeah!" he replies. "You're the one with the ponies, right?"

I am caught off guard. So he *has* been paying attention! Just because he hasn't answered my emails doesn't mean he hasn't been reading them. I let him get away with calling them "ponies."

"I'm writing a book," I inform him. "Your song…" I am so nervous I blank the name and have to flip to the song list in the liner notes to get the title. "…*One Prairie Outpost* is my theme song for that project."

I'd begun writing my manuscript shortly after the 2007 concert and the purchase of *Indian Summer*. That particular song is significant because of the line *"scene after scene passes by my life"* and the final chorus: *"One Prairie Outpost you are how I feel, alone in a flatland 'tween the dream and the real. The irony, ask me, 'where have you been?' I don't know, I don't know, because I don't know where to begin."* It expresses how I felt about taking on the writing of my own story.

"That sounds very cathartic," Barry says. "When is your book going to be published?"

"I have to finish it first, but I do have a literary agent who is very interested. So maybe in a few years. You'll still be playing then?"

"Oh yeah, we'll be around," he says.

"Hey," I begin, after some insignificant chatter, recognizing that I need to bring the conversation to a close. The floor behind the counter is elevated, and Barry is well over six feet tall, so I'm gazing up at him.

"I realize I have one of those unforgettable faces…" I start, but I only get that far when he reaches out spontaneously and cups my face gently in both of his huge hands. I am not sure how to react as I am caught totally by surprise. Somehow I manage to falter through the rest of my sentence. It takes all the concentration I have left. I think, *I hope,* I manage to maintain eye contact. "…and I just want you to know that when you play in Seattle you'll always have a familiar face in the audience."

He withdraws his hands.

"You coming to the show tonight?" He asks.

"Oh yeah. In fact, we need to get back downtown."

"Great! See you there."

"You bet."

On my way out the door, the remaining members of the band sign the inset as well. In hindsight, I feel bad that I hardly spoke with them, but I'd felt like I'd taken up too much of the band's time already and they are still strangers to me.

Ian tells me that my conversation with Barry was holding up the line and some people were getting disgruntled. I don't much care. I practically float back to the monorail.

The floor of the Showbox is densely packed by the time we arrive. I try to shoulder my way in on the right side of the venue (stage left) and am met with a harsh response from a blond woman.

"Hey, we've been standing here a long time!" she snaps, but as she turns to look at me she stops abruptly, exchanges a glance with her friend nearby, then looks away. It is how someone might react if they'd been bumped from behind and turned to make an angry comment like "watch where you're going" only to see it's an old man in a wheelchair.

"We can share the space," I reply halfheartedly, even as I notice her reaction. But she and her friend aren't listening. Her look and the mutual reaction of her friend indicate that they have dismissed me as someone they can't interact with normally, as if they've concluded I am mentally incapacitated.

Slightly embarrassed by their initial hostility and then abrupt disregard, I realize they do have a point. I had been gently elbowing my way into a dense area and had reached the limit as to how far I could proceed. So I return whence I'd come:

stage right, about four people back wedged alongside a railing. This is the side Terry plays on, referred to by the fans as "stage Terry." I am still close enough to be seen from the stage. Ian is watching from the elevated bar and my friend is standing behind me.

I smile to myself, considering the sacrifice many of these people have made. They have stood literally for hours, packed on the venue floor in front of the stage. They either didn't know about or gave up the opportunity to see the band at the record store just so they could be a sardine with a center stage view.

The band emerges to the roar of the crowd. Barry plays to his whole audience, not just those directly in front of him. During the second or third song, (*Changeless* in case anyone wants to know), he comes over to our side of the stage. I hold up my right arm, waving furiously to be noticed. Barry's eyes meet mine and I see his face change in recognition and he smiles broadly at me as he sings. The line of the song is *"I will not wait until the end, for my applause for you my friend."* He starts his applause motion as he sees me, cupping them around the microphone, and from my point of view it seems as if the gesture mimics the way he cupped his hands around my face back at the record store. His recognition of me is undeniable. My friend sees it too and thumps my back with excited congratulations of his acknowledgement.

I made an impression and I will not be forgotten. Likewise, Barry's unexpected reaction made an indelible impression on me.

Chapter Fifty Seven
"With the Band"

I often think back on what Barry's motivation was when he took my face in his hands. Compassion? Surely not pity. Does it matter? It was impulsive and wonderful. I am not a touchy-feely person, but that contact was magical. My friend teases me about Barry "laying on hands," yet I cannot help but feel that there was some sort of connection made that day. The power of a human touch should not be underestimated, especially when it is unanticipated. I wonder if he had any idea the effect it would have. It blew me away.

It sure helped in solidifying my devotion to that band.

I see Carbon Leaf again that fall at a special performance put on by the radio station on which I'd first heard their music. After the show, the band comes out to mingle even as the audience is rapidly departing. Terry, whom I've learned is the gregarious one, is the first one out and is immediately swarmed so I back off to wait for an opening. I spot Barry coming out. No one seems to be flocking to him so I approach him instead.

"I have something I want to ask you," I begin.

"Walk with me," he replies

He puts his arm around my shoulders, which at his stature is easy to do. I hesitantly return the gesture, putting my arm loosely around his waist, which at my stature is where it ends up. His shirt is cold and clammy from sweat, but I am so flattered at his familiarity that I don't let that bother me. We walk up toward the bar, chatting briefly. I am still in what I refer to as "the giddy teenager" stage, so I'm probably talking a mile a minute and an octave or two higher. It's a wonder he can understand anything I say. Maybe he can't and is just being polite. My friend is impatient to leave since she has to work the next day so I keep my conversation short.

I manage a quick hug and a very large *thank you* to Terry before departing. Terry's been especially kind to me without being patronizing so I feel particularly indebted to him.

In the car on the way home, my friend laments "you could have at least introduced me to Barry."

"But you weren't there," I responded guiltily.

"I was right behind you."

I ponder and the memory of her standing off to one side waiting seeps back into my brain.

"Oh, I guess you were. Sorry."

It was like tunnel vision. My whole attention was on him to the exclusion of all else. I didn't even realize she was there.

The following January, on the way to an Icelandic horse related meeting in Virginia, Ian and I detour to North Carolina to catch another performance by Carbon Leaf. Ian has by this time been won over by the band's talent and musicianship. Meanwhile, I have discovered that they use volunteers to run their merchandise booth, so despite having paid for tickets I sign Ian and I up to help them out. This means we are entitled to some interaction with the band before the show. I make a point of introducing myself to the members whom I'd brushed off in Seattle the previous summer.

"Oh, sure, I remember you," says Jason, the drummer.

"Oh, OK," I reply, a bit incredulously. I secretly feel guilty because I'd had to make a concentrated effort to not only remember the names of the bass player and the drummer but to look at photos so I could remember which was which.

Yet they all know me. Not only do they remember the face,

but most of them remember my name as well. And they remember *where* they saw me.

Yet at the same time I revel in this experience, I chide myself for caring so much. I am generally not an autograph seeker, and I can't bring myself to stand for hours basically immobilized by a crush of people just so I can be right next to the stage. Admittedly, right next to the stage is where I like to be. I've been able to secure that location at Billy Joel concerts back when you could get good seats merely by being first in line when tickets went on sale. My concert experience is enhanced when I can be up close and personal because not only do I get a close-up view of the performance, but that's where I can potentially be noticed.

Ian and I have since attended a number of Carbon Leaf's shows, volunteering at the band's merchandise booth at the majority of those. So while I am always excited to see them, my comfort level has increased. The embarrassing fan-girl giddiness has mostly faded and I've graduated from adoring fan to enthusiastic supporter. Yet while I consider myself a friend of the band, I don't fool myself into believing that any of the band members are my friends. My goal is to be reliable, to do good work for them, anticipate how we can help, and exercise the common sense to stay out of the way when necessary. It matters to me that the band members think of me and Ian in a positive way and are glad to see us coming.

For all the people I expose myself to during the hours I've worked in the merchandise booth, I've hardly had anyone overtly react to my appearance. I've noticed that one or two wait for Ian to assist them even though he is busy and I am available, but they do not refuse when I call them over. Perhaps being "with the band" gives me immunity. Many people think that I work for Carbon Leaf, so by association I am under an umbrella of acceptance. Not only do I feel useful and productive because I am making a positive contribution to a band I respect and admire, but I also feel secure in that setting. Working for the band in that capacity has become an escape for me, and on the rare occasions when I need to get away from other realities, I've been known to seek them out, especially when I think I can be useful to them.

I have no doubt my appearance helped make me more memorable to the members of Carbon Leaf and to the other bands and artists I've become acquainted with. Prior to a show for which Ian and I are allowed in early, I point out another benefit to Terry.

"All I have to do is walk around and make sure the venue staff see me and understand that I belong here. Then I can come and go as I please and nobody bothers me."

Too bad my face doesn't have a switch so I could flip it to *on* when I want to be noticed, but then to the *off* position when I would rather be invisible.

Yet for those who spend any time around me, the *off* button has already been activated. After spending some time around me, people just don't notice anymore. They don't even have to like me to reach this stage. It is merely a matter of familiarity.

I wonder if people use my face to describe me to others who don't know me. I do. I send a photo if I need to meet someone somewhere who has never seen me. But those who know me might not even think to do so because they've forgotten what I look like.

Chapter Fifty Eight
Out of Sight, Out of Mind

As I walk out of the vet's office, a young blond boy stares at me. I say "hi" to him in an effort to diffuse his curiosity and show that I am a real person. He shyly says "hi" back to me. *Good.* Often engaging with children diffuses their overactive curiosity, because they are forced to interact with me as another human being.

His mother and an older boy who is taller but otherwise a spitting image are still at the car. I say hello cordially as I pass. The mother carries a small terrier wrapped in a towel. She returns the greeting politely but without enthusiasm.

However, as I walk by, I can hear the youngest boy behind me.

"Did you see her?" he says.

I bristle and slow my step, but wait. I want to be sure…

"Did you see her?" he repeats. I imagine that he is talking to the brother. Then a third time. Then "did you see her face?'

That's it. I turn.

"Yes, he probably did see me," I reply earnestly. "If you have a question for me you are welcome to ask."

My tone is harsher than I mean it to be.

"OK," comes the quick reply from the mother, as if cowed or perhaps embarrassed by the confrontation. I grimace. I wasn't talking to her. It is not she who should be responding.

"I am not deaf," I add curtly, and wheel to return hastily to my truck.

Some days, some hours, some minutes, I handle it all right. Others, like now, it throws me off. Hurt, angry and near tears, I start the diesel and pull away, but I cannot take my temper and frustration out in my driving. Not while I'm hauling horses.

You would think after 40+ years I'd be used to it.

I claim that I don't want sympathy. But sometimes, just sometimes, maybe I do. More than that, I want to be looked upon and treated like a normal human being.

I want parents to raise their children to respect others and not meekly turn away when confronted with their own poor child-rearing practices. Instead of staring at me, *just ask*. Instead of talking behind my back, at least wait until I am out of earshot.

Was my response the best way to handle the situation? Likely not. But ignoring it and walking away would have been either. Ideally, I would I hope that the mother at least talked to her son about the situation, but in this case I somehow doubt it. So the child learns nothing.

Ideally, I become the educator. My tone would be more inviting as I seek genuine understanding, one human to another, that differences are OK. But alas I am human, and opportunities will be missed due to the fickleness of mood.

My facial features make me distinctive, yet I recognize that I am not completely unique.

A young man enters the Boys and Girls Club one afternoon while I am working. I cannot help but notice his face since the distortion is much more extreme than mine. One ear is on a different plane, reminding me of a Picasso painting. I've seen him before because his brother comes to the club, and it has been explained to me that he had been in a car accident. Given that everyone says that about me, I wonder how true it is.

He stands in the doorway. I figure he is just looking for his brother so though I glance his way I do not approach him. The ultimate hypocrisy is that I actually feel a little *uncomfortable* approaching him! Are we supposed to have some affinity because we both have different faces? It's not like we have a secret society with a secret handshake that makes us kin.

When he continues to stand there, my obligation as staff takes over. I approach him and look him in the eye.

"Can I help you?" I ask cordially. At least I have learned from how I like to be treated how to react to him. *As if nothing is different.* Eye contact, don't stare, don't search his features.

"Is Brad around?" He inquires. He seems positive and upbeat.

"Not in here," I reply. "Probably in the computer lab or outside. Have you looked there?"

"No, I'll do that, thanks," he says.

End of conversation. I have a twinge of regret not addressing him sooner, because apparently he was waiting for me to do so.

Is my reaction to him the same way that people react when they see me? What degree of difference does there need to be for people to have this kind of reaction? Am I a hypocrite, or am I excused because I am not looking at myself all the time and therefore unless I am somehow reminded I don't view myself as *different?*

My drug Addict eX-roommate (MAX) would come home sometimes and say something like "you know, you're not so bad-looking. I saw this woman on the ferry whose face was burned and she was really fat. She looked way worse than you." Like it was flattery. Like it was supposed to make me feel better about myself because there are people out there uglier than me.

Which brings up an interesting point. I consider myself lucky. Overall, I've had a pretty ordinary life. Physically and mentally, I am fully functional aside from what could be considered normal wear and tear. I completely understand that there are people who look physically normal who are way more messed up than I am. Others have had life experiences way more traumatic and emotionally devastating. There are people with visible physical differences far more challenging than mine who would gladly trade for my face. And I am grateful that my overall health is reasonably good.

These are the types of things I remind myself whenever I am tempted to wallow in self pity.

When I am asked, yet again, if I was in a car accident or if I suffer from Bell's Palsy, I have my oft-repeated reply ready:

"No. Tumor. At birth. I have been like this all my life. I know nothing different."

And I realize how lucky I am for that, too.

"Now that so much time has passed and medical technology has advanced so much, have you considered having more work done on your face?" This is a question I hear often. "After all, they're doing face transplants now."

"My understanding is that face transplants involve soft tissue over an internal structure that is pretty much intact," is my rehearsed reply. "My internal structure is not. Plus there is no practical way of replacing the nerves or activating the muscles, since I have a paralysis issue."

I'm not saying *never* because never is a word that has a tendency to come back and bite you in the butt. However, it would take a lot of convincing, because there are a couple of things that stop me from contacting a plastic surgeon and asking if anything more can be done. Primarily, nothing comes without a price, as prior experience testifies. Surgery is painful and results are never guaranteed. In my case, seldom did any procedure meet my expectations.

Besides, I've reached a certain degree of acceptance. I've gotten used to who I am, and I am afraid that changing my face would change my identity.

I consider myself lucky that I've had all my life to adjust. I suspect it would be worse to have once looked normal, perhaps even beautiful, and then in a single fleeting instant have that turned upside down, or twisted as the case may be. To peel off the bandages and have a scarred, asymmetric visage looking back from the mirror. These people are thrust into a new way of life and they become sudden, unsuspecting victims of how the world views physical imperfection.

"That guy keeps staring at you," my niece Jessica informs me as we're finishing up lunch in the mall.

"Oh, really? I hadn't noticed."

"I want to go up to him and punch him in the face."

"That's not necessary," I assure her. I don't know whether to be amused or annoyed. I don't even bother to look over to see who she is talking about. I figure he's not worth my time or attention.

A similar conversation occurs several weeks later.

"It really bothers me the way some people stare at you," says a close friend after we'd been shopping together.

"I didn't notice them," I reply. Kudos to those who have stared at me and not been obvious about it. Out of sight, out of mind.

Yet the abrupt reminder troubles me. I know my friends and family love me and mean no harm, but nonetheless it seems strange to have those I care about call this to my attention. Honestly, I think I prefer oblivion. After all, there is some truth to the notion that what you don't know can't hurt you.

I have come to understand that most of my life experiences are not unique. When my sister Lynne dies unexpectedly in June of 2007, a part of me dies with her. I am flooded with condolences, which I am grateful for, but at the funeral and the wake, I look around at her friends and realize that many of them knew her better than I did. I lost a sister whom in many respects I barely knew, but they lost a dear and intimate companion and friend. I often wonder if I should have reached out more and done more with her on a social level. If I should have tried harder to be more of a friend rather than just a sister. *Just a sister.* But I remind myself how different we are. Were. And I realize through the perpetual grieving process that being a sister is enough.

I am not the only one to experience this loss or to contemplate the *what ifs* of having done things differently. We all know or will know people who are sick or dying. We all know or will know people who have died unexpectedly, ripped from our lives without warning. The older I get the more I seem to be surrounded by it. We look forward to each coming year with hope that it won't be as bad as the previous, but each new year has its own tragedies. We have to hope that enough good things happen to counter balance the bad.

Our individual experiences shape who we are. It is how we deal with those experiences and how we confront each day that make us different from one another. It's easy to wallow in sadness and tragedy, or to wonder "why did this happen to me?" Such dejection can morph into self-pity, which can be OK, for awhile. I'm fine with feeling sorry for myself on occasion. When loss or any kind of emotional pain affects us, we each deal with grief in our own way. But at some point we each have a choice to make about how we want to go forward with our life.

Make the best of the cards you are dealt. Maybe I'm fortunate to be holding a face card.

Resources for People With Facial Differences

Publications:

Facial Shift; Adjusting to an Altered Appearance, by Dawn Shaw. http://www.facinguptoit.com/books/

Changing Faces, by James Partridge. http://changingfaces.org.uk/

The Church of 80% Sincerity, by David Roche. http://www.davidroche.com/

Full of Heart: My Story of Survival, Strength and Spirit by JR Martinez. http://jrmartinez.com/

Life with Scars by Brady Armstrong. www.rarecases.com

Internet

Changing Faces' self-help guides https://www.changingfaces.org.uk/Adults/Self-help-guides

Facing Forward, Inc. http://www.facingforwardinc.org/

AboutFace http://www.aboutface.ca/

Phoenix Society for Burn Survivors http://www.phoenix-society.org/

Moebius Syndrome Foundation http://moebiussyndrome.org/

Friending the Mirror webinar series http://www.facinguptoit.com/webinar/

BStigmaFree http://bstigmafree.org/

The Adults with Facial Differences Networking Community on Facebook

The Physical Differences Support, Discussion and Advocacy Group on Facebook

The Craniofacial Conditions – Support & Resources Group on Facebook

Acknowledgements

Allan Prell for getting me started on this rewarding yet often painful journey.

Doug Chandler and Marilyn Thuener for slogging through the first draft with me.

Wendy Harrington for providing encouragement and introducing me to my editor.

My editor Debra Ginsberg, who totally redirected my approach to the material for the better.

My husband Ian Shaw for being supportive in oh, so many ways.

My brother Brian Daugherty, my parents Richard and Adrienne Daugherty, and my late sister Lynne Wilson. Thanks for being there for me and for filling in gaps now and then.

The musicians in my life, especially Ian McFeron, Alisa Milner, Michael Tolcher and the members of Carbon Leaf: Barry Privett, Terry Clark, Carter Gravatt, Jon Markel and Jason Neal, for giving me encouragement, inspiration, motivation and support. Sometimes knowingly, many times not.

Tami Mathisen, who gave me a compass direction and showed me a star to steer by as the project neared its end.

To everyone's ears I bent talking about this project, thank you for at least pretending to be interested.

To everyone in the book and everyone else I know who isn't, thank you for being part of my learning experience, whether you reside solely in my past or continue on into my future.

About the Author

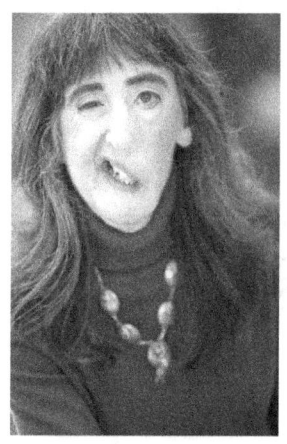

Professional motivational speaker Dawn Shaw understands adversity and embodies resilience, which she believes is the key to bully-resistance.

After *Facing Up to It*, she's published two additional books: an eBook exclusive titled *Friending the Mirror; Changing How You See Your Reflection*, and *Facial Shift; Adjusting to an Altered Appearance* (available in eBook and print formats). She has hosted an online video series, also titled *Friending the Mirror,* in which guests share their personal stories about coping with physical differences. Archived episodes are available on YouTube and via Dawn's web site www.facinguptoit.com. In November of 2016, she presented a TEDx talk titled *Beauty Is an Inside Job*, also available via her web site.

When not writing or speaking to youth or adult groups about such topics as developing resilience, accepting and embracing differences and the importance of not allowing *what others think* to affect one's identity, Dawn indulges in her affinity for live music, attending concerts primarily by independent rock bands with Ian, her husband of over 20 years. She also runs a small horse farm in western Washington, which is home to several well-loved cats and dogs and an ever-changing number of Icelandic horses.

Thank You Offer for Readers

Special Offer!

Visit www.facinguptoit.com to download an audio version of her Kindle eBook *Friending the Mirror*, a how-to guide on developing resilience by finding beauty through happiness.

Dawn Shaw is a Professional Motivational Speaker.

In her signature speech, Dawn emphasizes the importance of not allowing *what others think* to affect how we see ourselves. Youth and adult audiences alike are drawn in by her openness in sharing her personal stories about living with a facial difference. Her direct, engaging and entertaining style compels confidence in her audiences, leaving them more accepting of differences in both themselves and others.

What people are saying about Dawn's presentations:

"Dawn helps students develop understanding for and appreciation of people with differences instead of making fun of them."
—Andrew Smallman
Director, Puget Sound Community School, Seattle, WA

"Dawn's talk far exceeded expectations. She blew the veil off a sensitive topic and helped give a much better perspective on people who may generally appear to be physically different."
—Victor Ulsh
Program Chairman, East Bremerton Rotary

Visit http://www.facinguptoit.com/speaking/ for information, testimonials and booking.

To see Dawn's TEDx talk *Beauty is an Inside Job*, visit Dawn's web site.

Want to read more? Look for *Facial Shift; Adjusting to an Altered Appearance*, available in print and eBook formats, and her Kindle eBook, *Friending the Mirror* at http://www.facinguptoit.com/books/

Find Dawn on Twitter @facinguptoit and Facebook www.facebook.com/facinguptoit

www.ingramcontent.com/pod-product-compliance
Lightning Source LLC
Chambersburg PA
CBHW071854290426
44110CB00013B/1143